Managing Herpes

Managing Herpes

HOW TO LIVE AND LOVE
WITH A CHRONIC STD

by *Charles Ebel*
&
Anna Wald, M.D., M.P.H.

AMERICAN SOCIAL HEALTH ASSOCIATION
RESEARCH TRIANGLE PARK, NORTH CAROLINA

American Social Health Association, Research Triangle Park, NC 27709-3827

Book Design: Colleen Carrigan
Layout: Teresa Smith Perrien
Illustrations: pp. 11, 35, 40, 41, 42, 43—Mike Dulude

Library of Congress Catalog Card Number: 2002104394
ISBN 0-9716349-1-2

CONTENTS

CONTENTS

CONTENTS

ILLUSTRATIONS

PREFACE

At the National Herpes Hotline, the phone rings all day, every day. "Can you tell me if this is really herpes?" the callers want to know. "Do you think I got this from my lover?" "Is my doctor right when he says I'll have it for the rest of my life?" "Will I ever be able to date again?" "Can I have healthy children?"

Since 1979, through the hotline and other programs, the American Social Health Association (ASHA) has been helping tens of thousands of people each year find answers to questions like these.

This book draws on ASHA's experience in education and patient advocacy and also on the experiences of many who have contacted ASHA for information or who have participated in surveys, support groups, and focus groups. To protect confidentiality, we have used fictional names. But the anecdotes you will find here are based on the stories of real people who have chosen to share them with us.

Likewise, the medical information and tips reflect the expertise of many fine scientists and health educators who have collaborated in guiding ASHA's herpes work over the past two decades. This work includes local support groups and a quarterly journal, in addition to the National Herpes Hotline and educational material such as this book.

We hope this book offers some immediately useful guidance in managing genital herpes, and we hope also that it will prove a valuable source for future reference on herpes and other sexual health issues. But the best part is this: If you have further questions, ASHA will be there to help.

Charles Ebel
Anna Wald, M.D., M.P.H.

ACKNOWLEDGMENTS

As *Managing Herpes* goes into its Third Edition, it is again appropriate to acknowledge past and present members of ASHA's Scientific Advisory Committee on herpes: Lawrence Corey, M.D., Stephen Straus, M.D., Gray Davis, Ph.D., Zane Brown, M.D., Sevgi Aral, Ph.D., Joan Wiebel, R.N.C., Edward Hook, III, M.D., Lawrence Stanberry, M.D., Ph.D., Mauricio Vargas-Cortes, Ph.D., Robin Saltzman, M.D., and James Farr, M.D.

It is also fitting to acknowledge ASHA colleagues who provide leadership to the Herpes Resource Center program and great service to the public. These include Leigh Jolley, Joanne Grosshans, Mitch Herndon, and Michael Stalker.

A special thanks to Rhoda Ashley, Ph.D., for sharing data from several of her studies on diagnostic tests. Thanks as well to Nicholas Puryear for his thorough copyediting of the entire manuscript and to Teresa Perrien for typesetting and cover design.

1

THE NEWS

"I had been managing on my own as a single parent for nine years," says Carolyn, *"and I'd decided to pursue what I thought might be a promising relationship with a man I'd recently met. Several weeks later, there I was at the gynecologist's office, hearing that I might have genital herpes. The doctor gave me some printed material and a prescription, and sent me next door to deliver the culture test to a lab for an accurate diagnosis. I was holding back tears, wanting to hide from everyone, somehow feeling they were all staring at me. When I got to my car, I drove straight home and read the material over and over, hoping to find I had something else."*

For some, a diagnosis of genital herpes doesn't come as a complete shock. They may have had a partner who had it or may know enough about its symptoms to make an educated guess. Many first learn they have herpes when they seek medical attention for some kind of symptom in the genital area, though they might not have suspected that herpes would be the explanation. For a few, a herpes diagnosis is the unpleasant surprise result of a blood test taken as part of a broader work-up for sexually transmitted diseases (STDs). Whatever the circumstances, it's safe to say nobody likes getting diagnosed with genital herpes. Some may see it as a relatively minor issue—the inevitable price of being sexually active—yet still not good news. For others, it's a traumatic event, capable of causing a range of intense emotions.

One of the factors that gives herpes the potential to cause distress is the fact that it's a sexually transmitted infection. Growing up in American society, many of us come to view an STD like gonorrhea or syphilis—or, more recently, herpes—as something strange and horrible that happens only to those who have done something wrong. People who deserve trouble in their lives. People of bad morals. Attitudes about STDs vary depending on religion and a number of other cultural factors, but many of us have a hard time accepting the fact that we have an infection spread through having sex. It's often something about which we're taught to feel ashamed—or at least embarrassed.

Is this a reasonable attitude? Certainly few people would go out of their way to acquire an STD. Most of us would prefer to remain free of illnesses, whatever they might be. But the fact remains that all of us get sick during our lives. All of us are exposed to, and ultimately infected with, a host of bacteria and viruses that pose challenges to our health. Some of these germs are spread through the air or food or through contact with household objects that have been in some way contaminated. Some are spread through close physical contact with another person, including sexual contact.

Most of us are astonished to learn that infections spread through *sexual contact* are among the most widespread in our society. In fact, researchers believe that only the common cold surpasses STDs in the number of people affected. According to a recent study by the Kaiser Family Foundation and the American Social Health Association, there are more than 15 million new cases of sexually transmitted disease every year. *That's 41,095 people, newly infected, every day!*

When you think about it, the fact that STDs are so rampant shouldn't come as such a huge surprise. After all, people in all walks of life do have sex. It's as much a part of our biological make-up as eating and sleeping. And when we have sex, we sometimes pass a variety of common germs back and forth. One of the most common, it turns out, is herpes simplex virus (HSV), the cause of genital herpes. This particular infection is a fact of life for at least 45 million people in the U.S.—one in five persons over the age of 12. An increasing number of us understand how prevalent herpes is, but most, ironically, do not translate this information into a sense of personal risk. Despite what we know "on paper," we tend to see herpes as something that will happen only to someone else.

It's normal to feel some embarrassment about getting any sexually transmitted infection, even to feel that this condition somehow separates you from your friends, or changes the way you will interact with them. But getting an STD is hardly a rare event. And as you can see, getting herpes puts you in rather large company.

All this is not to say that you don't have a right to your feelings if a herpes diagnosis has caused you distress. Herpes is for all of us an unwelcome guest, and one of the things about it that is so distressing is that it's probably a lifelong guest. Often the first questions we ask the doctor in that fateful office visit focus on getting rid of it. "What do we do about it? What drug can I take? What's the cure?"

The answer, as you probably know by now, is that medical

science as yet has no cure for genital herpes. There are a number of medications that can help to control herpes, although none can wipe it out entirely. Some people choose to rely on these to keep herpes under control, while others come to feel that they don't need any medicines. Researchers, of course, are still hard at work, and the search for new drugs continues. Several types of vaccines are also in development.

In the meantime, it's important to remember that, *with time*, most people find herpes is not the catastrophe it might seem to be at the start. The physical and emotional distress of herpes usually peaks early on, often in the first few months.

The experience of millions of people shows that herpes does not have to be—and usually isn't—a major, life-changing event. Depending on the circumstances, and the type of symptoms involved, it often does require a process of adjustment—in our view of ourselves, in our relationships, and sometimes in the way we approach our physical health and well-being. The first step is to gain a better understanding about herpes and the issues it raises in our lives.

By opening this book, you've already taken that first step.

2

A VIRUS
IS A VIRUS
IS A VIRUS?

Genital herpes is caused by a virus—herpes simplex virus (HSV). In order to understand herpes more fully, it's important to start with the big picture and go over some key facts about viral infection in general. This chapter doesn't deal directly with many of the practical issues you may be facing if you're just recently diagnosed with herpes, but stay with it: A grounding in some of the basics here may help you later as you try to answer some of your own specific questions about genital herpes.

You may or may not remember much about viruses from high school biology, but you've been coping with them for most of your life. There are literally hundreds of families of viruses and thousands of individual types. Rhinoviruses, for example, are the frequent culprit in the common cold. Influenza viruses cause the respiratory ailments known as the flu. And a host of enteroviruses cause the intestinal disorders that almost everyone copes with from time to time. Other infectious diseases caused by viruses run the gamut from measles to hepatitis to AIDS.

HERPESVIRUSES: THE FAMILY TREE

Some people find the term *herpesvirus* confusing. Spelled out as one word, *herpesvirus* actually refers to a family of viruses with certain traits in common. This family includes Epstein-Barr virus, the cause of infectious mononucleosis ("mono"); varicella zoster, the cause of chickenpox in children and shingles in adults; and herpes simplex, the cause of cold sores on the face as well as genital herpes. (See table below.) The recently discovered herpesviruses—HHV-6, HHV-7, and HHV-8—may cause illness in some people, but research on these is still in its early stages.

HUMAN HERPESVIRUSES

HERPES SIMPLEX VIRUS, TYPE 1	HSV-1
HERPES SIMPLEX VIRUS, TYPE 2	HSV-2
EPSTEIN-BARR VIRUS	EBV
VARICELLA ZOSTER VIRUS	VZV
CYTOMEGALOVIRUS	CMV
HUMAN HERPESVIRUS, TYPE 6	HHV-6
HUMAN HERPESVIRUS, TYPE 7	HHV-7
HUMAN HERPESVIRUS, TYPE 8	HHV-8

As you can see from this family tree, most of us have had dealings with at least a couple of herpesviruses by the time we reach adulthood. Almost all of us, for example, are infected with varicella zoster as children. We suffer through the usual drudgery of chickenpox—the fever, the sores—until we pull through and shake the infection. Similarly, many of us have experienced a bout with "mono" sometime in our teens or early twenties.

Like all other viruses, a herpesvirus makes its way in the world by living in healthy cells. Once it gets a hold in the body, it finds a way to invade normal cells and disrupt their usual functions. The virus uses the machinery of the normal cell to produce more copies of itself, a process called *viral replication*.

Medical science has found ways to kill many types of bacteria and other disease-causing microbes. Antibiotics, for example, prevent bacteria from dividing and multiplying. Perhaps because many antibiotics are so effective, we have come to expect a pill that will rid the body of whatever troublesome infection we face.

But most viral infections, unlike bacterial infection, defy treatment—they can't be cured the way antibiotics cure strep throat. Scientists have found it more difficult to stop viral infections. The classic example is the common cold or the intestinal virus that takes us to the family doctor looking for relief. The usual response goes something like, "It's probably just a virus—there's not much we can do except to let it run its course."

In reality, a virus doesn't simply "run its course," tiring out and quitting by itself. Rather, it's our set of natural defenses—the immune system—that finally halts the illness brought on by viral invaders. The process may take days or weeks, but with the most common viruses the immune system eventually wins out, and the virus is eliminated. End of story.

Unfortunately, with herpesviruses the story has another chapter. The catch is that the herpesviruses find a way to retreat from the immune system and persist in the body without causing any symptoms. This ability to persist—to find a permanent hideaway—is called *latency*. Once established, latent herpesvirus infections are capable of remaining in a dormant phase, sometimes for long periods of time. Latent herpes infections, however, also are capable of becoming active again at unpredictable times. When this happens, the virus reactivates, begins to replicate, and sometimes causes symptoms of illness similar to those it brought on the first time. The majority of the herpesviruses—including HSV-1 and HSV-2—follow this pattern.

The most familiar example of this cycle of initial infection, latency, and reactivation is probably that of varicella zoster, which causes chickenpox. As children, almost all of us are exposed to varicella zoster and thus develop a case of those nasty little sores all over the body, along with fever and other symptoms of infection. In time, the sores heal and we recover. What's more, our bodies have perfected the strategy for an immune system attack on varicella zoster. So the next time we're exposed, we don't get sick—we have developed an *immunity*. It is nonetheless possible to have a flare-up of herpes zoster later in life, which is called *shingles*. This second episode is brought on by the virus that has been hiding away in the nerve roots inside our own bodies—not by exposure to someone else who is sick.

HERPES SIMPLEX VIRUS (HSV)

With this as background, let's look more closely at HSV and how it's going to affect you and your health.

To begin with, there are two distinct types of HSV. These look almost identical under a microscope and have many of the same properties. The chief difference between them is that they have marked preferences when it comes to where they live. HSV-1 prefers to live above the waist. It's best known as the cause of the fever blisters or cold sores that people get around the lips, mouth, and nose. HSV-2 prefers to live below the waist. There it can produce sores on the genitals that sometimes resemble cold sores. While the two types of HSV have *sites of preference*, as researchers call them, they are also somewhat adaptable. HSV-1 is capable of gaining a hold and causing trouble in the genital area. Likewise, HSV-2 can occasionally bring about cold sores on the face.

How It Spreads

HSV spreads from person to person through direct contact. Unlike common cold viruses that may pass through the air when someone sneezes, and unlike an enterovirus that might find its way to you on a contaminated piece of food, HSV generally requires skin-to-skin contact as a route of travel. It also requires a target area of skin that is vulnerable to its advances. Some types of skin cells—the soft skin of the genitals, for example, or the moist surfaces of mucous membranes such as in the mouth, vagina, and anus—offer relatively easy access for the invading HSV. The thicker skin of the arms, torso, and legs, by contrast, is too tough and usually can't be penetrated by HSV.

With these facts in mind, consider three very basic scenarios:

- A person with a cold sore caused by HSV-1 kisses someone on the mouth and spreads the virus. This causes the second person to get cold sores on the mouth as well.

- A person with genital herpes caused by HSV-2 has sexual intercourse with a partner and spreads the virus, causing the partner to develop genital herpes.

• A person with HSV-1 cold sores performs oral sex on a partner, causing the partner to develop genital herpes sores. In this scenario, we have genital herpes caused by HSV-1.

The spread of herpes is a complicated subject, and it's discussed in more detail later. For now, the important point to remember is that HSV spreads through skin-to-skin contact, from an area of skin where virus is present to a skin site that is susceptible.

Active and Inactive Phases: A Thumbnail "History"

What happens when HSV gets in your body? Once infected, the pattern and timing of events differ somewhat from person to person, but the basics remain the same. Once HSV gains a foothold, the virus begins replicating, invading the local nerve cells, and spreading. As we mentioned earlier, the defining event of infection is latency—the virus's successful effort to set up a permanent base of operations. With HSV, this process of latency occurs in the nerve roots. Having traveled the nerve pathways, HSV finds safe sanctuary in nerve roots called *ganglia* (see Figure 1). In cases of genital herpes, HSV retreats to the sacral ganglia, located near the base of the spine. In oral-facial herpes, HSV finds its way to the trigeminal ganglia, near the top of the spine. In these ganglia, the virus remains safe from the immune system and is capable of returning to an active state, though it can remain inactive for various periods of time.

The appearance of signs and symptoms during HSV's initial invasion is a tricky issue. The process of infection and latency requires only a few days. Therefore, the virus has become entrenched *before* a person might experience symptoms. Many people who develop symptoms will notice them within the first 10 days.

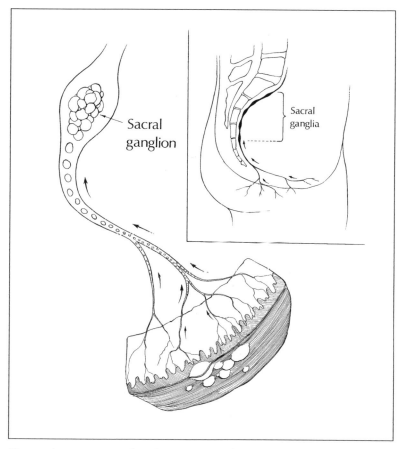

FIGURE 1. *HSV retreats along the nerves and finds sanctuary in the sacral ganglia, shown here.*

On the other hand, one's first encounter with HSV may cause changes so subtle that they aren't recognized. We'll discuss this in more detail in the next few chapters.

Beyond the initial infection and establishment of latency, there is also the prospect of reactivation. When HSV is latent, various biological events can cause it to become active and begin traveling the nerve pathways back to the skin. There it can cause signs and symptoms once more (or perhaps for the first time).

How Common Is It?

Some people are shocked to learn how widespread herpes simplex is. Researchers estimate that 66% of all Americans over the age of 12 are infected with HSV-1, most of which represents cold sores—oral herpes. Some people get an initial HSV-1 infection and have a bout with cold sores in childhood and then have no recurrences of the infection in their adult lives. Studies show that only about a third of those with latent HSV-1 report having had flare-ups with visible cold sores. HSV-1, then, is for the most part a commonplace and very benign infection. Only about 1 in 10 infected persons, or approximately 15 million, will experience recurrent oral-facial herpes several times per year.

HSV-2 is not as widespread, but it's hardly a rarity. Research data released in 1997 showed that 22% of Americans age 12 and older are infected with HSV-2, and the total number of people with genital herpes is estimated at more than 45 million. When we consider the population group of those age 18 and older, roughly one in five persons has HSV-2 infection.

If you're having trouble believing there are so many people with genital herpes, bear in mind that most don't know they have it. Researchers can test blood samples in a population to find out what percentage have HSV-2. When they interview those who test positive, *up to 90% say they have never had herpes symptoms!* In studies where these apparently symptom-free individuals are questioned further, a majority will recall some minor genital symptoms that they had never thought of as herpes. The other group holds to its initial testimony: no history of genital sores or the like.

What makes one person react so differently from another when infected with the same virus? Some scientists guess that these differences reflect variations in the individuals' immune responses; others suspect they center on the actual quantity of virus one is infected with, or on the particular sub-strain of the virus involved. As yet, however, researchers can't fully explain the huge variability in herpes symptoms among equally healthy adults.

THE BOTTOM LINE

To cut through all the science, keep in mind a couple of very basic facts:

First, if you have HSV, you have in your body a virus that operates, in most ways, just like dozens of other viruses you've carried around from time to time. The trouble with herpes simplex is that your immune system can't completely get rid of it. The virus can hide away and enjoy a lengthy stay through latency.

Second, you're not alone. The majority of adults carry around some form of herpes simplex, either type 1 or type 2—or both. They may not know it, because it may cause mild symptoms or no symptoms at all. Either way, however, with a latent infection like herpes simplex, the potential for viral reactivation persists.

So, medically speaking, herpes is neither an exotic nor an especially dangerous infection in the vast majority of people. We're talking about a "garden variety" bug. No more, no less.

3

THE STD YOU DIDN'T
KNOW YOU HAD?

⟨◎⟩

"My partner and I didn't want to be taking any risks in this new relationship," says Shelley, "so we decided we'd get HIV tests and get checked for STDs. At my clinic, when I asked about STD tests, they told me there's a new blood test for herpes and asked if I wanted that included in my STD screening. I said yes. Well, the result was positive for HSV-2. I was stunned. At first, I thought it had to be a mistake. I've never had this, I told them. Never had anything wrong sexually. But now that I've read more about it, I can see that herpes can be a sort of silent thing. Anyway, what I'm wondering is: What now? Do I need to do something about it?"

Most readers of this book probably have had symptoms of genital herpes, and the way they view it is colored by the physical reality of it. As new technologies take hold, however, it's likely that a significant number of readers are being diagnosed based on type-specific blood tests—tests that work in the absence of symptoms.

The most extensive study to date on the prevalence of genital herpes is called the National Health and Nutrition Examination Survey (NHANES). The method in this NHANES survey is to draw blood from 40,000 persons who represent a cross-section of the U.S. population, and test it for a variety of medical conditions. One of the tests employed identifies the presence of herpes simplex virus type 2 (HSV-2). The NHANES results for 1991 showed that 22% of the U.S. population over the age of 12 had HSV-2 infection. Even more surprising than this, however, was the percentage of those who are apparently symptom-free. When interviewed about a past history of genital herpes symptoms, a full 90% of those infected with HSV-2 gave no history of symptoms.

As you can see from the figure below, the proportion of genital herpes cases in which there are symptoms that cause someone to seek medical care is quite small. But there is more to the story.

A number of smaller studies using these specialized blood tests have made similar findings: that is, 80% to 90% of persons who have HSV-2 infection report no history of symptoms. In some of these smaller studies, however, researchers were able to

History vs. No History

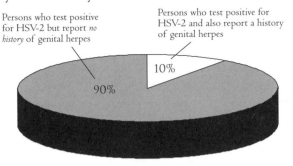

The NHANES survey shows that only 10% of those testing positive for HSV-2 are aware that they have genital herpes.

develop a more in-depth profile of these apparently asymptomatic subjects. For example, they spent time teaching the study recruits about herpes, and in particular used photographs to show examples of the types of signs and symptoms than can be associated with genital herpes—some of which are quite subtle. This educational process yielded another surprising result: After a few months, up to 62% of those who initially reported no history of symptoms were reporting that they could now recognize some form of herpes. The figure on this page shows an overlay of this data on the NHANES data. It suggests that while only 10% of those with HSV-2 have obvious recognized symptoms, perhaps as many as 70% to 80% have unrecognized symptoms, and the remaining 10% to 20% may be truly asymptomatic.

In any case, before we delve into more detail describing symptoms, treatments, and how the virus behaves over a long period of time, it makes sense to address the question: *What sort of*

Unrecognized vs. Asymptomatic Infection

This figure illustrates the phenomenon of unrecognized herpes: While 90% of those testing positive for HSV-2 initially give no history of herpes, the majority of this group is likely to recognize herpes symptoms when educated.

herpes information is relevant to the person who hasn't had any symptoms—or at least, hasn't had any symptoms he or she is aware of?

In general, most of the scientific research on herpes over the past half-century has been conducted in people who do have symptoms. However, since the mid 1980s, as scientists perfected HSV blood tests, we are beginning to learn much more about the large number of people who either have no symptoms or who have subtle, unrecognized symptoms. The findings of this research suggest that on some counts HSV operates the same way in persons with mild or unrecognized symptoms as it does in persons with obvious recurrent infections:

• All persons who are antibody-positive for HSV have latent infections, as described in the last chapter. HSV has established a permanent base of operations in the nerve ganglia. For HSV-2 (genital herpes), this is most likely to be the sacral nerve ganglia.

• Many people who test positive for HSV-2 and never recall having symptoms actually do have very mild symptoms they can learn to recognize as herpes.

• Whether a person experiences obvious symptoms or not, HSV-2 does reactivate from time to time, traveling the nerve pathways. Thus, there are times a person with unrecognized herpes might transmit herpes to a sexual partner.

There are, of course, differences as well. Readers who have been diagnosed solely on the basis of a blood test may find the description of *first episodes* to be completely unfamiliar. Likewise, the observations here on patterns of recurrences over the long term may not apply. Those who have never had herpes symptoms may also take a very different view on the need for—or role of—treatment.

Equally important, our description of the emotional and psychosocial issues associated with herpes might also ring false. If you feel that this book overstates the psychological impact of a herpes diagnosis, that is perhaps because the existing literature on herpes is drawn mostly from those with symptomatic recurrences. As we suggest in Chapter 1, in our limited experience with serologic testing thus far, a positive result for HSV-2 is seldom welcome news, but most people adjust well over time.

As we have constructed this edition of *Managing Herpes,* we have attempted to keep in mind the fact that readers may have broadly diverse experiences with genital herpes. All the same, if you have been diagnosed based on a blood test, like Shelley in the opening vignette, you may find yourself wanting to skip over some of the material. However, we suggest that you read with special attention a number of specific chapters:

> Chapter 5, "Recurrent Genital Herpes: The Long Run"— Because so many people can learn to recognize subtle signs and symptoms of herpes recurrences, the description of symptoms in this chapter may be helpful. In addition, there is information here about HSV's cycle of dormant and active phases.

> Chapter 6, "How Is Herpes Spread" and Chapter 7, "Who's To Blame"— These chapters address the confusion that people might have about how they have

acquired herpes and concerns about when and how they can transmit herpes to sexual partners.

Chapter 8, "Patient and Provider" and Chapter 9, "Treatment Options"— If you have never yet had symptoms, you may see little purpose in seeing a medical professional about herpes, but the time may come when you do need treatment or professional consultation. The first of these two chapters outlines some of the benefits of getting professional care and offers suggestions on how to approach the issue with your provider. The second explores current treatment options.

Chapter 10, "Sorting Out the Emotional Issues"— If getting a positive test result has been traumatic, this chapter may be a useful tool in thinking through the next steps.

Chapter 12, "Herpes and Your Sex Life"— A high percentage of people who have genital herpes are concerned about the effect it will have on their sexual relationships —and especially about the risk of transmission. This chapter explains the risk of transmission in couples and explores options for reducing that risk.

Chapter 14, "Herpes and Pregnancy"— The risks of transmitting herpes to a newborn—though a rare event—should be understood by every couple in which one or both partners have herpes. Men, too, should be educated on this topic, because the highest risk of neonatal herpes arises in couples in which the expectant mother acquires herpes during pregnancy.

IN THE END, the person who as yet has had no symptoms may have an easier time managing herpes as a health issue. But there are still several key aspects of this viral infection that will be worth your while to understand well.

MANAGING HERPES

4

THE
FIRST EPISODE:
HSV'S INITIAL IMPACT

"I was shell-shocked over having herpes anyway," says Erik. "But I was also pretty sick. I had wet blisters on my genitals, I itched like I had poison ivy, and I felt really run-down, too. It was almost like mono, with a sore throat and swollen glands. I don't know whether I was depressed or just sick, but I also felt listless—didn't want to do anything. I just lay in bed most of the time, and missed a couple of days of work. When the medication kicked in, I could see the sores healing up and I started to feel better. But it was two weeks before all the symptoms were gone."

As we mentioned in the previous chapter, many people infected with herpes simplex virus (HSV) either have no symptoms or, more likely, mild symptoms that they don't recognize as herpes. But a significant number—perhaps a third—will have symptoms of the infection right from the beginning. For many, like Erik, the trouble begins with a very difficult period of illness called first episode. This is likely to last longer and to cause more discomfort and stress than symptomatic periods that might occur later.

THE IMMUNE RESPONSE

First episodes are capable of stirring up considerable trouble because the invading virus has the element of surprise. Your body's defenses are not prepared for herpes. It takes a while before the immune system can identify the invader and refine its weapons to combat HSV. As it does, your immune response will succeed first in slowing the invasion and finally in forcing HSV to retreat from the field of battle.

Unfortunately, this doesn't happen overnight. The body's natural defense needs careful coordination among various parts of the immune system. These include the cellular immune response (the work of lymphocytes and macrophages) and the humoral immune response (antibodies). Using a combination of defenses, your body will try to kill the virus as it moves from cell to cell, will get rid of cells already infected, and will try to protect cells that are still healthy.

As all this microscopic warfare is carried out, it may take several weeks before any progress can be made against the invading virus. But in the long run there is good news. After its initial struggle with HSV, your immune system will remain prepared for future encounters. For example, the body keeps on making the specific antibodies that cripple the virus, and they will work more quickly the next time HSV emerges from the nerve roots.

How long a first episode lasts will vary a great deal from person to person. Probably the most important factor is your prior history with HSV.

Let's say that you've never had either HSV-1 or HSV-2 before. Through sexual contact you become infected with genital herpes caused by HSV-2. This is not only your first encounter with HSV-2, it's your body's first glimpse at herpes simplex of either type. So the virus is able to replicate and spread before the body can mount an effective counterattack. The same scenario might occur with a first exposure to HSV-1 as well. In either case, because your immune system has no direct experience with HSV, the body takes time to marshal its forces, and the signs and symptoms of infection can be troubling.

By contrast, let's say that you're one of the many people who was exposed to HSV-1 as a child and has had the virus for years, whether you know it or not. At age 25, you become infected with HSV-2 through sexual contact and develop symptoms. Your immune system has seen HSV-1 before, but HSV-2 is a slightly different entity. Your natural defenses react much more quickly than in the first example, but they aren't able to keep herpes in check. Here, too, signs and symptoms often follow, though they're often not as dramatic as those in the first example.

In the scientific literature, these two kinds of first episodes are sometimes given different names. The first kind, in which a person has never had either type of HSV before, is often called a *primary first episode* or *true primary*. The second type, in which the person infected with HSV-2 is already infected with HSV-1, is called a *nonprimary first episode*. In this book, however, we will simply use the term *first episode* to describe any early symptoms resulting from initial infection with HSV of either type.

FIRST-EPISODE SYMPTOMS

If the process of infection is going to produce marked symptoms, these symptoms typically start within the first 10 days after exposure to HSV. Often the first sign of trouble is genital itching or pain, followed by a red spot or some other change in the skin on or near the genitals. Next comes the emergence of sores or *lesions*. (The scientific literature uses the term *lesion* to describe a wide range of abnormalities in body tissue, such as any break or irregularity in the skin.)

In first-episode genital herpes, lesions may appear in men on the penis and urethra, the scrotum, the upper thigh, or around the anus. In women, they are commonly found on the vulva (lips of the vagina), urethra, cervix, and upper thigh, or around the anus. The illustrations on pages 40–43 show these locations.

When first seeing a healthcare provider, people with first-episode genital herpes usually have several lesions in different places in the genital area. About half the time, these are followed by a new crop of lesions in the second week. All in all, first-episode lesions will cause pain or discomfort for an average of 9-12 days and will take two to three weeks to heal fully. Lastly, as in the case of Erik, up to one-half of patients with first episodes experience more generalized symptoms, such as fever, malaise, headaches, and swollen glands, especially the lymph nodes near the groin. These generalized or "systemic" symptoms are more common in women than men.

First-episode lesions often follow a predictable pattern, in which the lesions develop into fluid-filled vesicles that eventually form a crust and then a scab before healing completely. In addition to these "classic" symptoms, however, genital HSV infection can show itself in numerous ways. Lesions may be almost invisible to the naked eye or may look like a small pimple or insect bite, perhaps going unnoticed. Then again, they may be large and obvious, superimposed on a patch of red skin. Sometimes sores will be extremely painful to the touch; sometimes they will not. Because of their varied appearance, herpes symptoms sometimes are mistaken for heat rash, jock itch, or ingrown hairs. The wide range of symptoms and their similarity to other conditions is one of the major reasons why so many of those who have herpes don't know it.

When a first episode produces classic herpes lesions, health-care providers often diagnose the condition based on the appearance of the lesions and the flu-like symptoms that frequently go along with them. First episodes can also lead to a number of other complications. One is difficulty in urinating. Lesions in the urethra itself can make it painful to pass urine, especially for women. If you have this problem, experts recommend that you urinate in a warm bath to ease the pain of contact with undiluted urine. In a small number of cases, the infection might actually affect the nerves that control urination, causing the patient to start retaining urine, a more serious problem requiring special medical care.

Some patients with a primary episode also experience *aseptic meningitis*. This sounds serious but usually denotes only an intense headache. Meningitis brings with it a stiff neck and sometimes extra sensitivity to light or loud noises. For reasons unknown, this too is particularly common in women. In the end, meningitis that results from HSV resolves by itself and rarely recurs.

Though technically not a symptom, another potential problem with first episodes is the risk of spreading herpes to another part of the body. With first episodes there is more virus on the skin, and it persists for longer periods of time. Because the immune system hasn't yet set up a solid defense for herpes simplex, it's possible to spread HSV from one part of your body to another part during this period—a phenomenon called *autoinoculation*. This sometimes happens when a person touches a herpes sore and then quickly touches another part of the body, which can have the effect of transporting a small colony of virus to a new site where it has the chance to replicate and spread. One example of this would be the person who touches a genital herpes sore and then moves the hand to the nose or mouth. A herpes sore on the face can result.

Some studies suggest that autoinoculation occurs in up to 10% of people with a primary episode, but is less common with other first episodes. After the immune response to herpes is fully established, autoinoculation is no longer an issue.

Lastly, the classic herpes lesions of a first episode may be susceptible to *superinfection*. In other words, the herpes lesions might become infected with fungus or bacteria, just as a cut in the skin might become infected. In women this may take the form of a vaginal yeast infection.

THE EMOTIONAL SIDE

The long list of symptoms is important to people with a first episode of genital herpes, but physical discomfort is only one piece of the problem. The American Social Health Association (ASHA) has heard from hundreds of thousands of herpes patients over the years, and the weight of evidence from these contacts suggests that the first episode of genital herpes also brings on the most intense emotions. Behavioral research and in-depth surveys also suggest an emotional impact that peaks in the first few months after a herpes diagnosis.

In a 1991 survey, for example, ASHA found that more than half of the 3,000 respondents noted feelings of depression, isolation, and fear of rejection during their initial outbreak. At the center of these feelings, people worried about the potential impact of herpes on their most intimate relationships. They experienced fears about the ways that herpes might change their sex lives. Some began to feel differently about themselves. Of equal importance, however, the survey also showed that these concerns diminish over time for a great number of people. The potential distress caused by herpes, including its sexual impact, will be discussed more fully in Chapters 10, 11, and 12.

WHAT YOU CAN DO

If you're experiencing your first bout with genital herpes, you're facing a host of issues and important personal decisions, such as whom to tell and how. Many of these questions are explored in detail in later chapters. The most immediate issues, meanwhile, are probably medical. Here is a brief list of steps that may help to keep the pain and anxiety of a first episode to a minimum:

- If you haven't already seen a doctor or other qualified healthcare professional, do this right away. With symptoms such as fever, headache, and swollen glands, you have every reason to seek a professional consultation. In particular, find out for sure whether you do indeed have herpes. For this, you often need a laboratory test, since there are other infections that can cause symptoms similar to first-episode HSV. Some patients try to diagnose themselves and later regret it, always wondering if it's really herpes.

• A number of diagnostic tests are available (see Chapter 16), some more accurate than others. Find out which test your doctor has used, and if possible, find out whether your symptoms are caused by HSV-1 or HSV-2.

• Discuss treatment options (Chapter 9). Antiviral drugs such as acyclovir or related compounds, such as famciclovir or valacyclovir, can hasten the healing process in first episodes, sometimes by several days. Treatment also dramatically reduces the duration of systemic complications, including meningitis.

• For added help with the pain and discomfort of herpes lesions, consider taking a quick warm bath a couple of times a day. Some people say these provide excellent temporary relief. After the bath, be careful to dry the infected area gently with a soft towel, or use a hair dryer on the low setting. Keeping the area clean and dry relieves discomfort and can speed healing. The use of topical creams and ointments, on the other hand, can actually make matters worse. Avoid hydrocortisone creams and consult your doctor before using any over-the-counter products.

• Take good care of yourself. You need rest, good nutrition, and relaxation to get well fast. Having herpes may raise some emotional issues that cause additional stress; try to put these worries on hold. The bottom line is that you're sick and you will get better soon. It may be easier to tackle some of the emotional issues a little later.

Both medically and psychologically, the first episode is in many ways the toughest challenge that HSV poses. Getting through it in the most positive way requires a variety of resources. These include competent and sensitive medical care and solid factual information. Beyond everything else, it's crucial to remember that the first episode is most likely the worst that HSV can throw your way.

5

RECURRENT GENITAL HERPES: THE LONG RUN

"It was about two months after my first episode," says Leslie. "Things were pretty much back to normal in my life, and I was hoping that I wouldn't have any more trouble with this. One week I was working late a lot and having trouble sleeping. I ended up feeling kind of run-down, and a couple of days later, the herpes came back.

"I remember being really upset about that second outbreak, and obsessing about it, checking myself all the time. That probably made matters worse, but even so, the sores lasted less than a week. And other than some itchiness, I felt fine.

"It turned out that I had about four or five outbreaks that first year, all pretty much the same. I didn't do anything special about them, because they weren't that much of a bother. Later the outbreaks got milder, but I still had about the same number each year."

If you're in the midst of a first episode, the very word recurrent may give you a feeling of dread. The prospect of going through this again is not a happy one. But don't think the worst: Recurrences of genital herpes are usually very different from first episodes and much less troublesome.

While Leslie's story is a familiar one, the specifics change for every individual. You may have only one or two herpes flare-ups in your whole life. You may have one or two each year. In some years, you may have a great many more. What happens in each case depends largely on a number of variables. Most, like the genetic make-up of your particular immune system or the sub-strain of virus you were infected with, are completely beyond your control. But some you can influence by the way you manage your health.

LATENCY

To understand the mechanism of recurrent herpes, let's discuss further the ability of herpes simplex virus (HSV) and other herpesviruses to hide away and persist in the body. Immediately after infection with HSV, a person may experience signs of illness (first episode) or may have no symptoms at all. Either way, the immune system will attack HSV and eventually force the virus to retreat.

Specifically, after the initial episode of genital herpes, HSV will move away from the skin surface and travel along the nerve pathways to the sacral ganglia, the nerve roots at the base of the spine. There, it goes into an inactive phase. As we explained in Chapter 2, the virus's ability to hide in this way and establish a permanent presence is called latency. During its inactive phase, HSV does not make more copies of itself (replicate) or move within the body. One analogy might be an army that retreats to a safe place and sets up a base camp. HSV's base camp in the ganglia is safe from the surveillance of the immune system.

REACTIVATION

When latent HSV does become active, it begins to replicate. To take our army metaphor further, we might think of active phases as times when the army will send out raiding parties to travel the nerve pathways towards the skin. Here the army

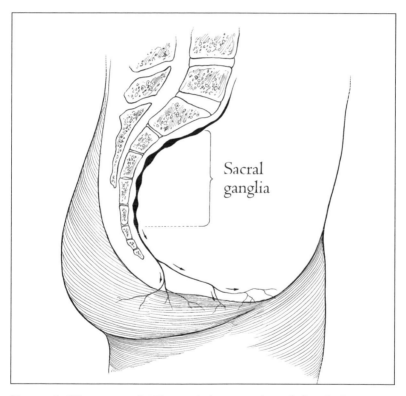

FIGURE 2. *When reactivated, HSV travels the nerve pathways back to the skin surface. Reactivation can cause the virus to reach the skin or mucosal membranes at many different sites in the genital area.*

becomes vulnerable to detection and counterattack, but it always has its base camp when it retreats.

Traveling the pathways of the nervous system in its active phase, HSV returns to the surface of the skin. There it can cause ulcers, sores, bumps, or other symptoms of genital herpes. This is often called *symptomatic* herpes, meaning that either the patient or the doctor has some physical evidence that HSV is again stirring up trouble. The medical literature uses the term *viral shedding* to denote the presence of active virus on a skin or mucous membrane surface during these times.

Latent herpes simplex also can become active and travel the nerve pathways *without* causing signs and symptoms of illness. In

**STAGES OF RECURRENT GENITAL HERPES
AND THREE POSSIBLE PRESENTATIONS**

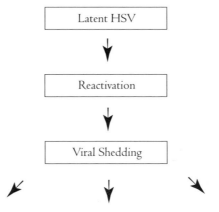

1. No signs or symptoms   2. Prodrome; mild symptoms   3. Classic lesions

the medical literature, this phenomenon has been called a number of things, including *asymptomatic viral shedding* and *subclinical shedding*. Here, when we use the term *asymptomatic shedding*, we mean the presence of virus on the skin or mucous membranes in the absence of symptoms. (In strict usage, *symptoms* refers to any marker of disease—including not only visible lesions but subjective feelings such as burning or itching. Therefore a person who experiences itching, for example, *would not* be asymptomatic.)

RECURRENCES WITH SYMPTOMS

Cases in which reactivation causes sores or other skin lesions are usually called *recurrences* or simply *outbreaks*. Here we will use the two terms interchangeably.

Most people who have a symptomatic first episode will have recurrences. With recurrences, people may experience a wide range of symptoms, some of them very subtle. As with first episodes, there are certain classic symptoms worth mentioning.

Prodrome

First, many people notice an itching, tingling, or burning sensation in the genital area before they see any visible signs of illness. These sensations are called the *prodrome*, and they can serve as a kind of early alarm system, warning that an outbreak may be on the way. Prodrome involves irritation along the nerves affected by HSV. Because nerve pathways connect in complicated patterns, this kind of irritation may lead to pain in the buttocks or the legs. Prodrome can last for several days but usually lasts less than 24 hours.

Other Signs and Symptoms

The prodrome is often followed by soreness or tenderness in a specific place, which in turn gives way to redness or skin irritation. Next, in many cases, ulcers or lesions resembling tiny blisters form on the skin. These can follow the same stages of healing described in Chapter 4, but fortunately, the lesions seen in a recurrence are usually fewer in number and heal more quickly. Studies report an average healing time of 4 to 6 days for untreated recurrences. Women tend to have more painful symptoms than men in recurrent herpes, but people of either sex very seldom have generalized symptoms such as fever, malaise, or fatigue.

Recurrent herpes usually affects the external genitals, less commonly reaching internal surfaces such as the cervix or the urethra. For example, recurrences produce evidence of virus on the cervix in only 12% of women, not the rate of up to 80% found in first-episode genital herpes.

We've already stressed that symptoms can vary a great deal from person to person. They can also change within an individual from one outbreak to the next, and certainly can change greatly over long periods of time.

Genital herpes can cause very minor signs and symptoms that are easy to overlook or, as we mentioned in Chapter 4, may be confused with other ailments. Herpes lesions may be as subtle as a pimple, a small break in the skin, or a tiny area of redness. Sometimes herpes sores look like small linear fissures and are mistaken for a yeast infection. Sometimes they may fall at the site of a hair follicle and be mistaken for an ingrown hair. Another example is minor lesions around the rectum, which are hard to see and are commonly mistaken for hemorrhoids. Not only are many of herpes' signs and symptoms subtle, but they frequently clear up quickly as well, perhaps taking only a day or two to disappear. Not infrequently, people experience prodrome and then have no lesions at all.

The wide variety of symptoms is the major reason that a visual diagnosis isn't always reliable. Illustrating the diverse symptoms and potential confusion associated with genital herpes, the table below was compiled by researchers at the Virology Research Clinic of the University of Washington. Patients presenting to the clinic with the initial complaints listed below were in fact diagnosed with genital herpes.

It's also worth noting that genital herpes symptoms don't always show up in the same place. A man might experience lesions

GENITAL HERPES SYMPTOMS MAY BE CONFUSED WITH . . .

In women		*In men*	
Yeast infection	Allergy to . . .	Folliculitis	Irritation from . . .
Vaginitis	• condoms	Jock itch	• tight jeans
Urinary tract infection	• spermicide • elastic/panty-hose	"Normal" itching	• sexual intercourse • bicycle seat
Menstruation	Irritation from . . .	Zipper burn	
Hemorrhoids	• bicycle seat	Hemorrhoids	
Heat rash	• shaving • douching	Allergy to condoms	
Urethral syndrome		Insect or spider bite	

on the penis the first several times he has an outbreak, for example, and then discover herpes lesions on his buttock or upper thigh the next time. Overall, about 20% of people will have a non-genital herpes recurrence, and the buttocks and legs are the most likely sites for such recurrences.

The skin lesions of genital herpes vary in appearance as well as in location. The following illustrations offer just a few examples of common sites for herpes recurrences. Lesions often are more subtle than those shown here. Because lesions may be located in the perineal or perianal area, or on the inner thigh, they may be difficult to see.

FIGURE 3. *Fluid-filled blisters on the shaft of the penis, consistent with recurrent genital herpes.*

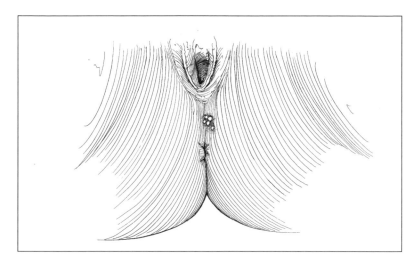

FIGURE 4. *Herpes lesions in the perineal area.*
FIGURE 5. *Herpes lesions on the buttocks near the anus.*

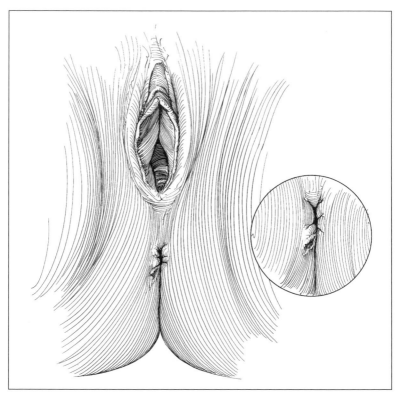

FIGURE 6. *A slight fissure (slit) near the anus. This is a common site for herpes lesions, which are sometimes mistaken for hemorrhoids.*

People sometimes find that the site of their outbreaks changes over time, and they worry that the virus might show up anywhere. It won't. A genital herpes infection is limited by the nerve pathways connected to the sacral ganglion. With genital HSV, signs and symptoms may migrate a few inches here or there, but they will remain in the same general area, below the

FIGURE 7. *Lesions of genital herpes on the buttocks. These are often thought to be "spider bites." They are sometimes misdiagnosed by healthcare providers as herpes zoster (shingles).*

waist. As noted earlier, there are instances in which herpes sores develop on the face, for example, during or after a troublesome first episode. These sores may result from autoinoculation; more commonly, though, they occur because a person has had a prior oral herpes infection. Don't jump to the conclusion that genital herpes has packed up and moved to the face on its own.

Post-Herpetic Neuralgia

One further note on symptoms: A small number of people with genital herpes report pain or discomfort in the general area of the healed lesions after the normal symptoms of a recurrence have ended. The term sometimes applied to this condition is *post-herpetic neuralgia,* meaning pain that extends along the course of one or more nerves. Post-herpetic neuralgia is frequently experienced by people with shingles (caused by the varicella zoster herpesvirus), and has been studied best in that population. Unfortunately, however, there is very little research on HSV-related neuralgia. The frequency of this complication remains unknown, and there are no widely accepted guidelines on treatment.

Based on what's known about shingles, people experiencing pain or discomfort following a herpes outbreak should regard HSV as being in its active phase during this time. Analgesics such as aspirin or ibuprofen are probably the simplest remedies available for the pain, but the antiviral medications discussed in Chapter 9 may also help to reduce the duration of post-herpetic neuralgia. Antivirals have been shown to reduce the duration of post-lesion pain in shingles patients by 50% or more. For people in whom post-herpetic neuralgia is linked with frequent recurrences of genital herpes, there may be value in using a daily antiviral medication to suppress the outbreaks and thereby lessen the problem of repeated irritation to the nerves.

How Likely Are Recurrences?

It's difficult to predict the pattern of recurrences in any individual case. There are, in fact, some people who never have anything resembling a herpes outbreak, with blisters and the like. The latest research suggests that as few as 10% of those with antibodies to HSV-2 recognize the infection—that is, when asked if they have ever had genital herpes, they say no. One would be tempted to assume, then, these persons do not have noticeable, recurrent symptoms. As we explained in Chapter 4, however, recent studies have shown that many of them do. In one such study, among a group of individuals who tested positive for HSV-2 but were unaware of their infection, roughly 70% to 80% learned to recognize recurrent symptoms after being educated about herpes by the research team. The bottom line: Most people with HSV-2 antibodies *do* have symptoms they can learn to recognize as herpes. In some cases, these might be marked outbreaks; in others, they might be minor irritations that could easily be overlooked.

These are large generalizations, taking into account all the millions of people for whom herpes symptoms will never be bothersome enough to spur a trip to the doctor. But the experts have more specific information when it comes to people whose first episode brought noticeable symptoms. Because these people often seek medical care, researchers have been able to run studies in which the patients are monitored for many years, leading to several important observations.

Viral Type and Sites of Preference

Whether and how often you have recurrences depends to a great extent on which type of HSV you have. If your primary episode is caused by HSV-1, for example, there is a 50% to 60% chance you will have a recurrence in the first year. By contrast, if the primary episode is caused by HSV-2, the chance of a symptomatic recurrence in the first year is 90%. And perhaps more important, people with genital HSV-2 are likely to have not just one but several recurrences in this and following years.

Why is this? Researchers don't fully understand it, but they know that type 1 and type 2 have definite *sites of preference.*

Scientists suppose that each viral type is triggered by certain events or chain reactions that may be specific to the body site where they're found.

In any case, HSV-1 causes the overwhelming majority of oral-facial herpes, and a person with HSV-1 latent in the facial area is much more likely to have recurrent outbreaks on the face than a person with HSV-2 in the same place. However, HSV-1 does account for an increasing percentage of genital herpes infections—anywhere from 30% to 50% depending upon the population studied. In addition, a first episode caused by HSV-1 is just as severe as that caused by HSV-2. However, people with HSV-1 genital herpes are likely to have only a few outbreaks or none at all after the first episode is healed.

The site of preference for HSV-2 is the genital area. HSV-2 almost never recurs above the waist, but, as we've noted already, it's extremely likely to cause genital herpes outbreaks, not only in year one but in later years as well.

Long-Term Patterns

As with predicting the likelihood of recurrences, predicting their number and long-term pattern is very hard. Do outbreaks become less frequent after five years? Ten years? Do they become less severe? While medical science doesn't have a way to predict the course of herpes for any particular individual, researchers have been studying genital herpes long enough to make some useful observations about long-term patterns of recurrence.

A study published in 1999, for example, analyzed the medical histories of 664 people with recurrent genital herpes over a period of 1 to 18 years. Consistent with earlier studies, this analysis showed that patients with HSV-1 had the lowest recurrence rates—a single recurrence on average in year one and a fraction of that in subsequent years. Patients with HSV-2, by contrast, had an average of five recurrences per year in the first year.

Of equal importance, the number of recurrences per year appears to decrease over time in the majority of patients, especially those with HSV-2. Overall, those who were enrolled in the study based on a first episode of HSV-2 and who were followed for more than 4 years had a median decrease of 2 recurrences per year between years 1 and 5. Thus, a person with 6 recurrences in year 1 would be having 4 recurrences after year 5, and a person with 4 recurrences in year 1 would be down to 2 outbreaks after year 5. Some 25% of the study subjects, however, actually experienced an *increase* of at least one recurrence per year, illustrating that herpes is highly variable from one person to the next.

Earlier studies reflected some of this variability as well, and it's impossible to predict where any given individual will fit into this game of averages. Among other observations made in long-term studies: patients with longer lasting first episodes tend to have more frequent recurrences than those with milder first episodes. Recurrences in men were 20% more frequent than those in women in the first year of infection.

REACTIVATION WITHOUT SYMPTOMS

For many years, scientists thought that HSV had basically two modes. One was the active phase, in which an infected person clearly had lesions or marked symptoms of some kind. The second was the inactive phase, in which HSV was out of the picture and of no consequence.

As they learned more about the virus, however, researchers

discovered that HSV could become active and yet *cause no symptoms*—at least none the patient would be aware of. This phenomenon is the *asymptomatic* form of herpes described earlier in this chapter.

With truly asymptomatic herpes, there is neither discomfort nor a lesion that the patient can see, so we might be tempted to write it off as irrelevant. But when virus travels to skin sites or to mucous membranes, there is the possibility of *viral shedding*, which creates a risk of spreading herpes to others during sexual contact.

There are still unanswered questions about asymptomatic viral shedding, but much has been learned in the last few years. Researchers have studied people who have visible symptoms from time to time, asking them to test themselves daily between outbreaks. In these studies, several observations seem fairly consistent:

> • Asymptomatic shedding occurs in the vast majority of people who have and recognize recurrent genital herpes. For some people it happens on less than 1% of the days in a year; for others, it may happen on up to 10% of days or more. Overall, the average is about 4% of days.*

> • The amount of asymptomatic shedding is greatest in the first year after one acquires herpes—roughly twice as high as in year two.

*Author's Note: Figures offered here reflect rates of shedding as documented by positive culture tests. Higher rates have been reported with the less well-accepted polymerase chain reaction (PCR) technique, which detects smaller amounts of virus than culture tests.

• As with symptomatic recurrences, asymptomatic shedding is more than three times as frequent in those with genital HSV-2 as in those with genital HSV-1.

• Roughly half of all asymptomatic shedding occurs within seven days before or after an outbreak.

• The risk of asymptomatic shedding exists in everyone with genital herpes. While the frequency varies from person to person, someone with mild disease may shed as much virus as a person with severe infection.

• Asymptomatic shedding can occur almost anywhere in the genital region. As with all HSV reactivation, the virus follows the nerve pathways connected to the ganglion at the base of the spine. Especially likely sites of shedding, however, are the vulva and perianal area in women or the shaft of the penis and perianal area in men.

• The amount of virus present is similar to what is found during symptomatic outbreaks, and it's often sufficient to spread the infection to a partner.

In summary, what's most remarkable about asymptomatic shedding is that it appears to follow the major patterns associated with recognized outbreaks: It often occurs immediately before or after symptoms appear; it's more likely with HSV-2 than HSV-1; and it produces quantities of virus sufficient to cause transmission.

What about those who are diagnosed on the basis of a blood test but have no history of symptoms—how often do they shed virus? Research on viral shedding in those with no history of symptoms is a relatively new undertaking, but some observations can be made based on a study published in 2000. In this study, 53 persons with no history of recurrences were educated about herpes, asked to perform daily swabs of the genital area for laboratory testing, and followed closely by clinic staff for just over three months. Results from this group were then compared with 90 subjects who had a history of genital herpes recurrences. Analysis showed the following:

- Eighty-three percent of those who gave no history were found to have viral shedding during the study.

- After education and counseling, 80% reported having a symptomatic recurrence during follow-up.

- Those with no history of symptoms had 60% fewer symptomatic recurrences, and the recurrences were 40% shorter on average than those experienced by subjects in the other group.

- Overall rates of viral shedding (including both outbreaks and days with asymptomatic shedding) were lower in the group with no history, with virus present on 3.8% of days, versus 6.4% in the symptomatic group.

- Rates of asymptomatic shedding were similar in both groups.

What these findings suggest is that those who have HSV-2, as measured by a blood test, but never recognize any symptoms do in fact have phases in which HSV becomes active and causes viral shedding. In this group, however, most of these active phases take the form of asymptomatic shedding rather than outbreaks. Asymptomatic shedding accounts for about one-third of all reactivation in those with recognized outbreaks and roughly 80% of shedding in those with more subtle infections, so it's important to understand it. Researchers already have established that asymptomatic shedding, as well as shedding during recurrences, can be largely suppressed with medication. This is covered in Chapter 9.

WHAT TRIGGERS RECURRENCES?

Long-term patterns in the cycle of active and inactive phases also raise the question: What triggers HSV to break out of its dormant phase and become active again? Can outbreaks be avoided simply by avoiding these triggers?

Over the years, people with herpes have put forth many candidates as the trigger for recurrent herpes. These include sickness, psychological stress, fatigue, menstruation, and poor nutrition. Sun exposure—even the mildest sunburn—can be a trigger for HSV, as can irritation or friction at the site of infection. And some say that vigorous sex can cause this kind of irritation.

Few of these possible triggers have been closely studied by researchers, but some work has been done. Scientists have noted several types of outbreak stimulants in lab animals, among them: skin irritation at the site of infection, surgical trauma to the nerve or ganglion where the latent virus resides, and radiation.

Recently, very detailed studies have looked at the role of intense ultraviolet light on facial cold sores caused by HSV-1. In these studies, 70% of the subjects exposed to about two hours of midday sun developed herpes symptoms within a week. Subjects who used sunscreen were protected. The message for people who get cold sores is clear, particularly if they're sensitive to the sun. On the basis of a few small research studies, it seems that ultraviolet light may well have a similar effect in triggering genital herpes in those who have prolonged and direct exposures of the buttocks or genital area.

Menstruation remains prominent as a trigger factor in anecdotal accounts, but researchers have found no evidence of this in research studies.

Psychological stress has received a great deal of attention as a possible trigger factor. Over two-thirds of the respondents in ASHA's 1991 survey, for example, indicated that "stressful events contribute to herpes symptoms." This issue also has been examined by a variety of researchers, with somewhat contradictory results. The latest study on stress, published in 1999, suggests that there is not a relationship between short-term stress—say, a deadline at the office—and genital herpes recurrences. There was, however, a slight increase in risk of a recurrence associated with stressors lasting more than 7 days—for example, a period of anxiety about prolonged unemployment.

In any case, can you avoid triggers? From a strictly scientific point of view, outbreaks cannot be predicted with accuracy. No one will be able to identify the certain cause of every flare-up, and some people won't have a clue about any of them. At the same time, however, it appears that many people with herpes do begin to associate certain events or behaviors with reactivation.

Once identified, triggers can *sometimes* be avoided. If sunburn gives you a bad case of cold sores, there is always sunscreen, lip balm, and a hat. If outbreaks seem to be brought on by fatigue, maybe it's time to get serious about a quality eight hours every night.

Stress is perhaps a more troublesome category. There is little point for most of us in trying to create "stress-free" lives. In fact, even if we did, there is no proof that we'd be free from HSV reactivations. Nonetheless, it's widely accepted that managing stress through exercise or other activities can be beneficial to one's overall physical and mental health. It's possible, though not proven, that this may have some benefit in managing herpes as well.

Many triggers are not known or can't be foreseen. Others you may have good reason to suspect but can't do much about. The last thing you want to do is blame yourself for recurrences or try endless experimental strategies to avoid them. For some, this becomes another form of obsession.

If, on the other hand, you gain clear insight into your pattern of outbreaks, you may find practical ways of sometimes averting them. Over time your knowledge of your own triggers and your sensitivity to prodromal symptoms will likely increase. This information, in turn, is something you can use in a variety of ways, including taking preventive medications or taking precautions to lower the risk of transmitting herpes to a sexual partner.

THE BOTTOM LINE

The next few chapters of this book offer many ideas on how to manage recurrent genital herpes. But there are a number of points we've already covered that are worth emphasizing:

• Viral type is the most important factor influencing the course of recurrent genital herpes. Therefore, it's important to know which type you have. Chapter 16 explains which diagnostic tests provide this information.

• Statistical data show that those with HSV-2 typically have several recurrences per year while those with HSV-1 have few or none. However, there is great variability between individuals. Some people have only a few outbreaks each year, while others have many. The pattern is slightly different for everyone.

• The symptoms caused by herpes outbreaks may change over time. Sores might appear in one spot this month and several inches away three months from now. Some outbreaks may simply result in irritation or redness.

• Outbreaks are not the only concern with genital herpes. There are times when HSV reactivates in the form of asymptomatic viral shedding, and one can be contagious at these times. Like recurrences, asymptomatic shedding tends to be more frequent in the first year and more frequent in those with HSV-2.

• There is little hard evidence about what triggers outbreaks, but a great many people report that they associate certain stresses or behaviors with outbreaks.

6

HOW IS HERPES SPREAD?

"I was just diagnosed with herpes," says a caller to the National Herpes Hotline. "And I'm worried about giving this thing to someone else. I'm confused about how I got it, and I don't really know when I'm contagious."

Understanding how the herpes simplex virus (HSV) operates and what you can expect it to do inside your body are crucial pieces of information. But equally pressing is the issue of *transmission*. People want to know how they got infected with herpes— when, and by whom, and in what precise way. They also wonder when they're contagious.

This is one of the most complex aspects of herpes and one that usually takes a bit of study to grasp fully. It may be necessary to read this chapter and the next a few times before the information makes complete sense or before you can remember it all.

The first basic rule is that genital herpes spreads from one person to another through various forms of sexual intimacy, all of them involving direct body-to-body contact. We'll talk about these in more detail on the following pages.

Second, the possibility that herpes will be spread from one person to another exists only at times when there is viral shedding—times when HSV is present on a skin surface or mucous membrane.

These periods of viral shedding are often marked by signs or symptoms that herpes has reactivated and reached the skin, such as the classic herpes lesions. Or there may be very mild symptoms that clear up in a couple of days. It's also possible that the viral shedding caused by an active phase will be entirely asymptomatic and that you will be totally unaware of it. This scenario will be covered more fully later in this chapter (see the section titled, "When No Symptoms Are Present").

Of course, the most flagrant sign that herpes has become active is the presence of sores or some kind of lesion on the surface of the skin. We'll address this issue first.

WHEN SYMPTOMS ARE PRESENT

As an example, let's say you have two or three herpes sores on your genitals during your first recurrence. The sores are, in effect, little colonies of virus, and as long as you can see them, you should assume you have significant amounts of HSV present on the surface of the skin. If you have sexual intercourse while the sores are present, it's likely that your partner's genitals will come in direct contact with these sores. That would give the virus a chance to spread to your partner's skin and take up residence there.

The risk of infecting another person begins with the itching or tingling feeling that you get right before an outbreak. If you notice any symptoms of recurrent genital herpes—even the pro-drome—take it as a sign that the virus has found its way to the skin or to the mucous membranes usually affected. The risk continues as long as you notice *any* kind of symptom. If sores or other skin lesions are present, it's best to consider these contagious until they have completely healed. The tender new skin you see after a scab falls off might not be contagious, but caution is advisable: Asymptomatic shedding is more likely to occur within the first few days before and after an outbreak than at other times.

Herpes can be spread through other forms of direct skin-to-skin contact as well. Consider what can happen during oral sex. When a person with a cold sore on the lips has oral contact with a partner's genitals, the virus has an opportunity. Herpes can spread from the lips to the partner's genitals, causing genital herpes.

The direct contact that occurs during oral sex also can cause an infection in the facial area. Let's say a person engages in oral sex with a partner who has herpes sores on the genitals. Contact with those genital sores can give the virus a chance to spread to the person's lips or mouth, resulting in herpes infection in the facial area.

Sexual intimacy provides several possible ways in which active virus may have a chance to spread from a site of viral shedding to susceptible genital tissue or mucous membrane in a partner. We've specifically mentioned oral-genital sex. Other routes of transmission include penile-vaginal intercourse, penetration of the anus, and oral-anal contact. Even the rubbing of one body against another without penetration might give active virus a chance to spread, assuming the uninfected person is exposing susceptible skin in the genital area.

All of this can be a little confusing. People sometimes ask, for instance, "Now that I've got genital herpes, does it mean the virus is going to migrate all over my body and trigger cold sores on the lips?" They wonder if they're going to be spreading herpes when they touch someone or kiss someone. The answer to all of these questions is no. Herpes simplex will not relocate from your genital area to your facial area or any other part of your body unless you give it a lot of help. It can be spread from the genitals to a sexual partner's face in the way we have described, but it doesn't get up and move all by itself. Remember the rule of thumb: Herpes is spread through direct skin-to-skin contact with an area where virus is active on the skin.

You may be wondering why herpes seems to take hold only in the genital region or around the mouth. HSV has evolved to thrive in warm and moist environments, and genital skin like that of the vulva or penis offers the virus a suitable entryway. So do soft, moist surfaces such as the vagina, cervix, anus, and mouth. The thicker, tougher skin on the arms and legs, by contrast, is generally not hospitable to HSV. If by chance HSV is deposited on these parts of the body, it usually withers before it has a chance to find the nerve pathways and go about the complex business of making its permanent home.

Notice the word 'usually' in the last sentence. There are some cases where herpes does penetrate the tough skin of the hands or the chest, for example. But in these instances the process of transmission is helped along by some damage to the skin in question.

A good illustration of this principle is an HSV infection called *herpes gladiatorum*—what some call *wrestler's herpes*. In a number of cases, high school or college wrestlers have developed herpes sores on the chest or arms in the aftermath of a wrestling tournament. Why? Wrestling involves rolling around on the mat and grabbing the arms and torso of the opponent, all of which can be abrasive to the skin—even thick skin. Add to this the fact that wrestlers spend a good deal of time in tight embraces, and you can see that direct contact with a cold sore (or with saliva that contains HSV from oral herpes) might give HSV a chance to spread from one wrestler to another.

This happens only rarely, and the circumstances under which it has occurred sometimes involve a wrestler who is particularly contagious because he is having a first episode of type 1 herpes on the face. During this kind of outbreak, large amounts of virus might be present on the surface of the skin or in saliva, and lesions on the face are not uncommon.

Another scenario in which herpes can spread to thicker skin is *autoinoculation*. As described in Chapter 2, this occurs when someone touches a herpes sore—on the genitals, let's say—and then ends up sometime later with a herpes outbreak on the tip of the finger. The route of transmission is clear. Active virus from a sore found its way to the finger when the person touched or scratched the sore. The virus then managed to find some portal of entry—a cut or scrape, for example—so that it could travel the nerve pathways and set up shop in a different location, such as moving from the genitals to a finger. Autoinoculation seems to be most common when the site of new infection is another mucous membrane. (Sometimes people get herpes sores in the eyes, a subject discussed in Chapter 15.)

To keep this in proper perspective, don't forget that autoinoculation is relatively infrequent. It occurs almost exclusively during first episodes, when there are lots of sores and an unusually high dose of virus on the skin. It's estimated that autoinoculation occurs in about 10% of first episodes, but it's rare with recurrent genital herpes. The reason is that over time the body develops a strong immune response to the virus.

To sum up, the best advice is to regard the presence of pro-drome, sores, or any potentially herpes-related lesion as a sign that the virus is active and could be spread. Any kind of direct skin-to-skin contact with the sores or lesions creates a risk for the spread of the virus, but it's almost always *sexual* contact—genital-to-genital, oral-to-genital, or oral-to-oral contact—that causes new infections.

WHEN NO SYMPTOMS ARE PRESENT

Unfortunately, the HSV's active phase is not always marked by the presence of signs and symptoms. Chapter 5 describes the phenomenon of asymptomatic shedding, in which herpes re-activates and travels to the skin without setting off the usual alarm system. It's now clear from a number of studies that herpes can be spread at these times, in a process called *asymptomatic transmission.*

These are troublesome facts of life for people with herpes, because they complicate the issue of protecting a sexual partner from infection. Even those who don't recall ever having had symptoms face this risk of giving the infection to a partner. Nevertheless, there are a number of ways to approach this prob-lem of asymptomatic herpes, and the best way to begin is by understanding more about how it works.

In a general sense, asymptomatic shedding is somewhat similar to regular outbreaks: While herpes is in its latent phase, some event triggers a recurrence. HSV travels through the nerve pathways to the area where it usually causes symptoms, and finds its way to the surface of the skin or to a mucous membrane such as the cervix. Meanwhile, the immune system comes into play and thwarts the virus, stopping HSV's spread before any major lesions appear—but unfortunately *not* before there is risk of transmission.

Where is asymptomatic shedding likely to occur? In most cases, HSV can be expected to travel the same routes it does during a symptomatic flare-up, and virus might reach the skin anywhere in the genital area, including the sites where you normally have signs and symptoms during a noticeable outbreak. In particular, asymptomatic shedding is likely on the vulva and perianal area in women, and the shaft of the penis and the perianal area in men.

As discussed in the previous chapter, patterns of asymptomatic shedding mimic recurrences in a number of ways. Asymptomatic shedding is highest in the first year after acquiring herpes, and in general, rates decline slightly over time. Just as recurrence rates vary greatly between individuals, so does asymptomatic shedding. One individual, for example, may have shedding on only 1% of days; for another the frequency may be 15%. The average is approximately 4%.

Whatever the actual rate in your case, the hard part is that you won't know which days these will be. So when it comes to protecting a sexual partner, this is an issue that requires you to talk things through and make certain decisions as a couple.

Asymptomatic shedding may be somewhat unpredictable, but there are things you can do to control it. Researchers have found antiviral therapy has basically the same effect on asymptomatic shedding that it does on outbreaks. In particular, a daily dose of antiviral medication produced a 94% reduction in shedding in one study. The possible role of medication will be discussed in depth in Chapter 9.

OTHER ISSUES FOR TRANSMISSION OF HSV

An important concern for couples who would like to have a child is the issue of managing herpes during pregnancy and birth. In some cases, HSV is transmitted to a baby at the time of delivery if the mother has active herpes in the birth canal at delivery. This is a very rare event among the tens of millions of women who have genital herpes, and there are well-known precautions that can prevent it in most cases. All the same, herpes infections in a newborn can be life-threatening, and expectant parents often have very specific questions about what they need to do to ensure a healthy birth. They also wonder about the risk to an infant in the home if one or both parents have recurrent genital herpes. We've attempted to answer these questions in detail in Chapter 14.

Another frequent question centers on the spread of herpes from *things* rather than from people. Can you get herpes from a toilet seat, for example, or a dirty towel? The basic answer on the risk of getting herpes from inanimate objects like these is something along the lines of "generally impossible." The main reason for this goes back to our earlier discussion about transmission, about skin-to-skin contact, and about the likely places where herpes can take hold. If you rubbed a herpes sore against a towel, for instance, some of the herpes simplex virus could be deposited onto the towel. The virus may persist outside the body for several hours, but soon it begins to lose its ability to invade and colonize new cells.

Now take the example of the toilet seat and follow the rules of transmission. In order to spread herpes, a person has to be infected, to have active herpes, and to have virus present on the skin. Furthermore, the skin in question would have to come into contact with the surface of the toilet seat. Since people generally do not rub their genitals against toilet seats, a person would have to have active herpes on the back of the thigh or lower buttock in order to place virus on the seat. This is not the most likely place to have an outbreak.

Next, within a short time, a second person would have to sit on the same seat, making contact with the seat in exactly the same spot, thereby coming into contact with HSV. And would the virus find a hospitable environment there on the back of the thigh? Probably not. The skin there is thick, making it an unlikely target.

Often, the context for questions about non-sexual transmission of herpes is the concern about parent-child transmission in the household. For example, a mother has a history of herpes and worries about diapering her three-month-old baby or getting in the tub with a one-year-old. What is the chance that herpes will be spread from parent to child over the course of many years of casual household contact—from diapering to sharing towels? Frankly, these questions do not have clear-cut answers based on scientific data. There is not a single published case of HSV transmission via an inanimate object, and the most logical conclusions to draw from this fact is that casual household transmission is extremely rare or nonexistent.

Researchers, however, do acknowledge a *theoretical* risk of nonsexual transmission. A damp towel shared by two people showering together, for example, could hypothetically provide a means for the spread of herpes to the genitals if one person were having an outbreak and rubbed the towel on the site of infection before passing it to the partner.

Experts disagree about whether herpes is ever *really* spread in this way, but because it's theoretically possible, common sense dictates precautions. During active phases, don't share towels, underwear, or other objects that come into contact with herpes sores. In cases of facial herpes, the items to avoid sharing during active phases would be cups, toothbrushes, and razors. And if you touch a herpes lesion with your finger, take the precaution of washing your hands right away. Soapy water kills the virus.

PEOPLE WITH HERPES are likely to have a number of worries about spreading the infection to other people. It's natural to have these concerns. But sometimes people will become obsessed with risks that are either very remote or completely nonexistent. So, to put things in perspective, here are some overall guidelines.

- The greatest risk for spreading herpes comes when you have a herpes symptom—no matter how slight—and your partner's skin comes into direct contact with that area during sex. Avoiding this kind of contact is the first concern.

• If you have recurrent genital herpes, you will want to talk with your lover about the risk of asymptomatic transmission when you have sex during the times between outbreaks. See Chapter 12 for a full discussion of the different approaches that people take to prevent the spread of herpes in sexual relationships.

• If you're having your first-ever outbreak of genital herpes (or facial herpes), it's wise to be extra-cautious about hygiene. Avoid touching herpes sores, and if you do touch them, wash your hands right away with soap and water. Soap will kill the virus.

• If you are pregnant and you or your partner has a history of genital herpes, it's very important to inform your physician or midwife about this part of your medical history. If genital herpes becomes active at the time of delivery, your provider may need to take special precautions to protect your baby. This is discussed at length in Chapter 14.

• If you have a newborn in the household, take care to see that the child does not come in direct contact with herpes lesions. It isn't wise, for example, to kiss *anyone* if you have a cold sore on the mouth, but this is an especially important rule with infants.

The most critical issues for preventing transmission of HSV center on your sexual relationships. These will likely be among your leading concerns as you adjust to life with the herpes simplex virus.

7

WHO'S TO BLAME?

"It was a mystery," says Julia. "I remember being diagnosed with herpes and wondering where I got it. I didn't have a clue. I hadn't slept with anyone in months. So I called the two people I'd been with, and both said they'd never had herpes. They thanked me for telling them about it. That was it. I never figured it out. And I never knew if I gave herpes to anyone else. I still wonder."

If you've just experienced your first outbreak of genital herpes—or if you were diagnosed on the basis of a blood test—you, too, may be asking the question: Where did I get this?

Given that genital herpes is a sexually transmitted disease, it's natural for people to scrutinize their current sexual relationships in search of an answer. Often they seek to blame a current partner for infecting them, especially if it's someone they've known only briefly. If they have been intimate with one person for a long time, they sometimes come to believe that this partner has recently had an affair, developed herpes as a result, and kept it a secret. Whatever the scenario, suspicion and anger are common elements, and they're often directed at a person's current lover.

Are these suspicions likely to be well-founded? It is possible to get a genital herpes infection from one's current sexual partner, but this is not always the correct explanation. Julia's story doesn't offer enough detail for even an educated guess, but with a little room for embellishment we can suggest at least three possible scenarios:

'It Had to Be You'

Julia is single and dating, having recently broken off a relationship of two years with Jim. She's currently seeing Mark off and on, and two months ago she slept with him a few times. Later she developed a genital rash and went to the doctor, who now has diagnosed her with genital herpes.

Can Julia legitimately blame Mark? The circumstantial evidence is fairly damning, but in this example Julia actually had acquired herpes from her earlier boyfriend, Jim. Neither of them knew he had it, because he was one of those many millions who carry HSV-2 and never realize it. She never knew she had gotten it, because she had no obvious symptoms when she was first infected.

Now, years later, something has triggered a reactivation of the latent HSV. Julia has symptoms, and she's blaming Mark.

'It Had to Be Infidelity'

Let's keep two of the players, but change the details of the story:

Julia has been living with Mark for almost a year. She gets genital herpes symptoms and is diagnosed with it. She wants to blame Mark and so confronts him.

Mark says he doesn't have herpes—never had any STD or anything vaguely resembling herpes. Just as Julia suspects him, Mark now begins to suspect her. He knows that he hasn't been intimate with anyone else for more than a year. Now suddenly he is accused of having herpes. So he wonders if Julia has recently had an affair, has picked up this infection, and is simply afraid to admit it.

Well, Mark is wrong. It turns out that Mark does have herpes and did infect Julia. It's just that he didn't know he had it. He's one of those people who has very mild and infrequent symptoms, and he has never considered that they were related to an STD. For all practical purposes, he's being completely honest and above-board. But he does have genital herpes. And now Julia does, too.

'A LONG STORY'

Let's try one more variation:

Having broken off a relationship with Jim a year ago, Julia moves in with Mark. Two months later Julia comes back from the doctor with a diagnosis of genital herpes. She blames Mark; Mark blames her. Accusations of infidelity fly. Mark denies any history of herpes.

Then suddenly Mark, too, gets herpes. Julia is now fully convinced that she was right to blame him all along. Mark is equally convinced that Julia is at fault.

As in the first scenario, Julia actually had picked up herpes from her earlier relationship with Jim. But things have gotten really complicated now. Julia never knew she was infected until she just recently had her first outbreak. Meanwhile, she had infected Mark.

Everybody has herpes, and it all started with Jim.

IS REAL LIFE like this? It isn't always, but it can be. Each of these scenarios is quite plausible.

If there is appeal in a guessing game, tracing genital herpes infection can be among the most challenging of mysteries. Countless people with herpes have puzzled over the spread of HSV and posed hard questions: How could this have happened to me? Are you sure it wasn't a toilet seat? Who was the culprit? Was my spouse unfaithful? Did my lover know he had herpes and keep it a secret from me?

For the most part, the questions cannot be answered. HSV, it turns out, is a very crafty virus. Trying to figure out how it spreads raises a host of complicated issues: signs and symptoms, viral type, previous sexual history, prior infection with HSV, and so on.

The fictional scenarios presented here offer a glimpse at three critical reasons why it's hard to know who is to blame.

The first reason is that *you can have herpes and never know it.* Earlier chapters have gone into some detail about the evidence that up to 90% of all people diagnosed with HSV-2 infection based on screening tests say they have never had herpes symptoms. A small proportion of this group, as we've explained, probably are truly asymptomatic. Most, however, have mild symptoms they did not recognize as herpes. Either way, a large number of people get herpes and never know it, never think about it—never have any reason to talk about it or take precautions.

The second reason is that *you can get herpes and carry it around for months or years before you finally have a recognized outbreak.* Researchers believe that something like one in four people seeking care for their first outbreak have actually had herpes for some time. It's possible to have a very mild first episode and to assume that it's something else—a yeast infection or an allergic rash, for example. Then, seemingly out of nowhere, the person with a mild or unrecognized infection can one day face a troublesome outbreak and wrongly assume that genital herpes is a new problem.

A third possible cause of confusion is that *you can spread herpes even when you don't have symptoms.*

Studies have conclusively shown that persons infected with genital HSV have periodic episodes of asymptomatic viral shedding whether they have symptoms they recognize or not. So there are times when virus is present on the genital skin or mucous membranes. And that raises the possibility of spreading it to someone else during sexual contact. People who know they have genital herpes usually take some precautions to protect sexual partners, at least during known outbreaks. People who are unaware they have it, on the other hand, may see no reason to practice any form of risk reduction with their sexual partners.

Of course, asymptomatic transmission is a risk even for people with outbreaks that they do recognize as genital herpes. Sometimes a person might be careful to refrain from sex when symptoms are present and be unlucky enough to spread HSV to a partner during a period of viral shedding between outbreaks.

If all this seems a little overwhelming, be aware that it can be overwhelming for almost anyone—including skilled medical professionals. If you're trying to pinpoint the source of your herpes infection, you may well run into some dead ends. And it's likely that your healthcare provider won't be able to solve the mystery either.

Is there any way to know for sure? Can you get special tests that pinpoint the source? The path is not an easy one, but there are some facts you can probably establish with the help of a medical professional. With the right diagnostic test, for example, you may be able to determine whether or not you are having a first episode or a recurrence. The antibodies that a newly infected person produces to fight herpes usually will not be fully in evidence until some weeks after initial infection. Therefore, healthcare professionals can sometimes test for antibodies over a period of time to watch for a trend. A person newly infected with HSV-2 would have few or no antibodies to HSV-2 when blood was first drawn but would normally have a substantial level two to three months later.

Diagnosing a first episode versus a recurrence based on this evidence, however, is not as straightforward as it may seem here. Much depends on the specific signs and symptoms, the timing of the office visit, and the particular tests used to make the diagnosis. Some blood tests are useful for this type of detective work, and some are completely unreliable. It's possible that the test you want may not be available to you through your current healthcare provider or that the results will not be definitive. A detailed explanation of available tests will be coming in Chapter 16.

In any case, even if a blood test reveals that you are having a first episode, this evidence will not necessarily tell you *the source* of your herpes infection. As the fictional scenarios at the beginning of this chapter suggest, a lot depends on your own sexual history and a host of factors too complicated to explain in a book of this size. The moral is this: Don't be too quick to judge the situation. Figuring out the source of a herpes infection can stump even the best medical detective.

What's more, even if you are fairly sure about how you got herpes, it can be very wrong to assume that the partner in question was acting irresponsibly. There are indeed some people who know they have herpes and withhold this information from sexual partners. But there are many more who have no idea they themselves are infected, much less that they might be putting you at risk. In the end, understanding and forgiveness may give you more comfort than blame or vengefulness.

MANAGING HERPES

8

PATIENT AND PROVIDER

"My diagnosing doctor was not all that helpful," says Barbara. "He told me I had herpes and gave me some medication, but he seemed pretty unconcerned about the whole thing. He said most people just see it as an annoyance—something they 'learn to live with.' I was devastated. My mind was racing."

For most people, the issue of getting the help they need begins with their healthcare provider. The provider is often the first person we ever talk to about genital herpes, and the tone and content of that conversation often shapes how we perceive herpes and how we manage it. Ideally, if you already have been diagnosed with genital herpes, your provider spent enough time with you to answer your questions about the herpes simplex virus, its likely pattern of recurrences, and the options available for treatment. If you had questions about how you got herpes, perhaps these were covered during the office visits, along with questions about your risk of spreading it to others. If so, you have an exceptional resource in your provider—a person you may be able to turn to as questions come up.

In many cases, however, people newly diagnosed with herpes report frustrations about their healthcare experiences. Even if you normally get along well with your healthcare provider, a diagnosis of genital herpes can complicate matters. It's important to be aware of some of the potentially tricky issues in order to continue a positive working relationship with your chosen medical professional.

If there are troubles, they often start with the visit in which herpes is diagnosed. The diagnosis itself is tough to hear and tough to deliver. And, depending on the individual, the diagnosis can raise several issues of importance to the patient. In all fairness, it's very difficult for healthcare providers to cover all of these issues in one visit. With a waiting room full of patients, there isn't time to say or do everything the provider would like to. Beyond this, providers may feel that they aren't prepared to discuss some of the emotional aspects of herpes.

From the patient's point of view, it's often devastating to learn that the illness at hand is caused by a sexually transmitted infection. Worse still, it's a viral infection and will stay with you for life. This news raises a great many questions about herpes itself and about its potential impact on important relationships.

The medical information alone is complex. The first several chapters of this book, for example, cover most of the basics. But how many healthcare professionals have the time to cover those topics on a first visit, especially if they haven't had the chance to schedule an extended session? Beyond this, patients can bring up emotional issues for which the healthcare professional may not have ready answers. "What will this mean for my sex life?" "How can I tell my lover?" Some of the questions cannot be answered in simple black and white.

From the provider's point of view, time and the patient's

emotions are the most important constraints. Healthcare professionals often say they do their best to counsel patients on the key points but that patients' feelings of anger or disbelief sometimes stand in the way. A patient might be too upset to take in a lot of medical information—or might not remember many details later even if they were covered in a counseling session. Plus, with a waiting room full of patients, there isn't time to say or do everything the healthcare provider would like. Sometimes the best solution seems to be scheduling a follow-up visit. Even then, however, patients can leave feeling overwhelmed and confused.

There is also the problem of unrealistic expectations. We often seek health care assuming that all questions can be answered and all infections can be cured. But in reality medical professionals are not all-knowing or all-powerful, and herpes may force the issue. Faced with questions like "Where did I get this?" the healthcare provider may well have to say, "I don't know." Rightly or wrongly, this can lead to feelings of frustration and helplessness in the patient. And when it comes to the sexual or emotional impact of the diagnosis, providers may lack both the time or the specific training required.

Whatever the specifics of your situation, it's important to try to keep the lines of communication open. Patients should have a way to get answers, to get treatment if they need it, and to get advice on something that can affect their intimate relationships. If you feel you need some more time, you might try to schedule a follow-up visit to discuss your questions.

We know from interviews and from surveys that significant numbers of people with herpes voice complaints about their first visit and about the healthcare provider who first diagnosed them. In ASHA's 1991 survey, more than half rate this provider as "poor" or "fair" when asked specifically about the provider's performance in answering questions, giving treatment information, offering emotional support, and discussing a patient's sex life.

Worse still, a small number of patients report that their providers make them feel ashamed about having herpes and make remarks that assess blame—for example, comments like, "You now have to pay the consequences for what you've done." Another frequent complaint, voiced earlier from Barbara, is that providers overlook the importance of leaving patients with a sense of hope or empowerment. Instead they may seem to be saying, "There is not much that can be done." Either kind of experience can have the effect of closing the door on further discussion of herpes. It can keep patients from asking the questions they need answered, getting treatment for current or future outbreaks, and getting advice they may want on a fairly intimate matter. It sets a negative tone that is hard to change.

Even if nothing especially awkward occurred during a first visit, herpes can have a chilling effect on open communication. Herpes may be difficult to talk about when we're first diagnosed—even with a medical professional. And this can pose a barrier to seeking further medical help, making one reluctant to ask certain questions or request follow-up consultations. Unfortunately, this cuts the patient off from a critical resource.

Among the benefits of professional medical care:

CORRECT DIAGNOSIS: People who try to diagnose themselves often regret it later. For example, a recent study has shown that

20% of patients seeking clinical care for genital symptoms were given a false positive diagnosis of genital herpes—that is, they were told they had herpes when they really didn't. Underdiagnosis of herpes is also a common problem. A confirming laboratory test can make all the difference, and it can be useful information to have on your medical record. In particular, knowing whether you have HSV-1 or HSV-2 may be helpful in predicting the course of the infection and in protecting partners. (For more on diagnostic tests, see Chapter 16.)

ACCESS TO ACUTE CARE: Patients with a first-episode infection may be sick for a couple of weeks or more and often benefit from medication. The most effective medications are available only by prescription.

TREATMENT FOR RECURRENT GENITAL HERPES: For a variety of reasons, patients may wish to use medication for recurrent herpes. As we explain in Chapter 9, prescription medications may help to alleviate symptoms or dramatically reduce recurrence rates.

PREGNANCY: Women who have a history of genital herpes often need some advice about how to manage herpes if they choose to become pregnant. This advice relates not only to treatment but to the precautions that should be taken to avoid passing herpes to a newborn at delivery and immediately after. Management of herpes in pregnancy also is an issue for men with HSV whose partners are pregnant and have no history of herpes. (See Chapter 14.)

WHATEVER THE SPECIFICS of your situation, it's important to try to keep the lines of communication open. Patients should have a way to get answers, to get treatment if they need it, and to get advice on something that can affect their intimate relationships. It's important to remind yourself that strained or awkward relationships between the patient and the healthcare provider often can be repaired. If you feel you need some more time, you might try to schedule a follow-up visit to discuss your questions. However, if you are convinced you will not be comfortable seeking care for herpes with your current provider, there is always the option of looking for a "second opinion."

If you do feel it's time to look elsewhere for medical care, physicians with specialty training in gynecology, urology, dermatology, and infectious diseases may have more experience or technical training on herpes. On the other hand, it may be most important for you to have a clinician who will make you feel comfortable asking questions or who will be supportive emotionally, in which case a family practitioner or primary care provider may be the perfect choice. Much depends on the individuals involved.

You may be able to get a list of referrals from your local medical society or from a local herpes support group. If you have a university medical center or teaching hospital nearby, you can also reach the department dealing with infectious diseases and ask for a herpesvirus or STD specialist.

Another problem cited by people with herpes is a lack of continuity in care in today's large group practices and health maintenance organizations. You may work through the awkwardness of a first visit for genital herpes and get to feeling comfortable with one doctor or nurse practitioner, only to find that he or she isn't available the next time you need help. Do you make an appointment with someone else at the practice? Do you have to go through the hassle of discussing herpes again, your sex life again? Many people find this difficult. It's important to remember, though, that your health shouldn't take a back seat on account of shyness. Herpes may well prompt legitimate questions and concerns from time to time. You should feel entitled to raise them. People who take charge and get the answers they want seldom look back and regret it.

WHAT YOU CAN DO

• Inform yourself about herpes and make a list of the questions and concerns you need to raise with a healthcare professional. Many people find it's a good idea to bring a written list when you have the medical consultation.

• It may take persistence to get the answers you need, but don't be afraid to ask your provider for help. Knowledge and emotional support are tools that can help put you back in control. If you have trouble broaching the subject, you might take a few minutes to ponder and rehearse a script. You might say, for example, "I feel awkward bringing this up, but I've had a history of genital herpes and there are some things that I've been wanting to get advice on." If the questions involve your partner, you might arrange to bring him or her along when you see the doctor.

• Ask the provider to explain your treatment options. Even if you decide not to use medications, knowledge is power. Don't let yourself feel cut off from treatment just because your provider didn't bring it up the first time. As explained in Chapter 19, health insurance and managed care routinely cover antiviral medication for herpes, and with the increased competition among chain and on-line pharmacies, the cost of these drugs is often significantly lower than it was five years ago.

• If what you need is primarily emotional support, be realistic about what your medical professional can offer. Depending upon your personal situation, you may be best served by seeking out a friend or counselor or looking to other resources, such as the National Herpes Hotline or a local herpes support group. There is a list of ideas at the end of this book.

For some, these suggestions may beg the comment "easier said than done." Establishing good communication about herpes often takes a dose of hard work for both the patient and provider. Most experts stress three general points above all: Inform yourself; communicate your concerns and questions to your healthcare provider in an organized way; and don't be afraid to seek a second opinion if you're unsatisfied. The work might be hard, but it's a prescription you can write yourself.

9

TREATMENT OPTIONS

⟨◎⟩

"My outbreaks were frequent and troublesome," writes Teri. *"It wasn't so much because of the sores, which cleared up quickly, but because of symptoms like headache, tiredness, and muscle aches. It was like having the flu about once a month.*

"I finally went to my gynecologist and started a course of drug therapy that has changed my life. I take medication every day, and now I'm symptom-free, in spite of a very stressful, demanding job and an active sex life.

"So far, so good, I guess. But I wonder how long it's safe to continue with this medication over the long term? And I wonder if there is cure on the horizon."

FIRST-LINE ANTIVIRAL THERAPY

Like many other viral infections, genital herpes can be treated with a number of medications. There are now three antiviral drugs that have been shown to be safe and effective at easing the symptoms of genital herpes. In some cases, these drugs stop outbreaks altogether for as long as the medication is taken. As helpful as these drugs are, it's important to stress that today's antivirals do not cure herpes. They can't eliminate the herpes virus the way a specific antibiotic can knock out a specific kind of bacteria. Once a person is infected, HSV establishes latency and persists in the nerve ganglia. Today's drugs cannot prevent latency, but rather attack HSV and curb its spread at times when it becomes active and produces viral shedding. Researchers continue to look for new, more effective treatments.

ACYCLOVIR — Three prescription medicines are currently approved by the U.S. Food and Drug Administration for the treatment of genital herpes. The best known and most widely prescribed is acyclovir, sold under the brand name Zovirax® since 1982. Acyclovir is now available as a generic. It's actually a rather remarkable drug—one of the first to be effective against a virus without being toxic to normal cells. The scientist who led its development, Gertrude Elion, received a Nobel prize for her research.

Acyclovir works by attacking HSV's ability to reproduce. Like other viruses, HSV can move from cell to cell in its active phase, colonizing the cells as it goes and using them to create more virus. At the molecular level, the key to this process is the virus's genetic assembly instructions, or DNA (deoxyribonucleic acid). Acyclovir substitutes itself for one of the building blocks of the viral DNA and fools the virus into accepting an impostor. Once acyclovir has slipped into the machinery of the virus, the DNA chain comes to a halt.

For the patient taking the medication, this translates into a win over HSV, as viral shedding is brought to a standstill and symptoms abate. HSV, meanwhile, still has its safe haven—its base camp—in the nerve roots. In practical terms, a patient with a nasty first episode might normally have to wait three weeks before the skin lesions are healed and things have returned to normal. With acyclovir treatment, the length of the outbreak might be cut significantly.

In addition to acyclovir, people with herpes have a choice between two newer antivirals. Both are prodrugs, which means they have a kind of two-staged delivery. In stage one, you take the prodrug, which is then easily absorbed into the body. In stage two, the prodrug is converted by the body into the active medication.

VALACYCLOVIR — Valacyclovir (brand name Valtrex®) is marketed by GlaxoSmithKline. Valacyclovir is the prodrug of acyclovir, converting to acyclovir after ingestion. This process has the advantage of getting higher levels of acyclovir into the body. Most people absorb only 15% to 20% of acyclovir when they take it in conventional form, but taking the prodrug can boost absorption to the 50% to 80% range. In practical terms, valacyclovir's major advantage is less frequent dosing.

FAMCICLOVIR — Famciclovir (brand name Famvir®), now licensed to Novartis, is the prodrug of penciclovir. Famciclovir is more readily taken up by the body than penciclovir. It converts to penciclovir in the body, resulting in higher concentrations of the active drug in the body than can be obtained with the oral administration. Like acyclovir, penciclovir works by sabotaging viral DNA. Famciclovir also appears to have an impressive *half-life*, the length of time it remains active in the body. Like valacyclovir, famciclovir can be taken less often than acyclovir.

FIRST EPISODES

Oral antiviral medication is commonly used for patients having a first episode. Here, given the large amounts of HSV present, and given the immune system's lack of experience in fighting the virus, medication can have dramatic results.

Taken for 7 to 10 days, antiviral medication can shorten the duration of herpes symptoms (itching and pain, for instance) by 40% to 50%. It can reduce the length of time during which a first-episode patient is contagious—by 70% to 80%. And overall, it can mean a 30% to 40% decrease in the total time it takes for skin to heal. Not everyone has a painful first episode, but if you're suffering through one, these statistics may spell welcome relief. Dosages recommended for a first episode of genital herpes are given in Table 9.1, below.

TABLE **9.1. Recommended oral antiviral regimens for first episodes of genital herpes***

Name	Brand	Regimen*
Acyclovir	(generic)	400 mg, 3 times daily for 7–10 days*
Acyclovir	(generic)	200 mg, 5 times daily for 7–10 days*
Famciclovir	Famvir®	250 mg, 3 times daily for 7–10 days*
Valacyclovir	Valtrex®	1000 mg, 2 times daily for 7–10 days*

*Therapy for first episodes of genital herpes should be continued for 7–10 days or until all lesions have healed.

RECURRENT EPISODES

Does antiviral therapy work against recurrent genital herpes too? It can, and here patients face a choice between two kinds of treatment. The first, called *episodic therapy*, means using medication to halt or shorten an outbreak once it has started. The second option, called *suppressive therapy*, means taking medicine every day in the hope that it will short-circuit reactivations of HSV and prevent outbreaks from occurring.

EPISODIC THERAPY — In this approach, a patient begins taking medication at the first sign of recurrence and continues for five days. (It's called *episodic* because one treats the individual episode and then stops taking medication until the next outbreak.) The results of episodic therapy vary quite a bit from person to person, but large controlled trials suggest the time to healing is generally reduced by an average of one to two days. If taken at the first sign of prodrome, episodic therapy can prevent an outbreak from occurring in some cases. Viral shedding, the period during which there is potential for transmission, may be reduced by half. Duration of symptoms (pain, tenderness, itching, tingling) may be reduced by 15% to 20%. The recommended antiviral dosages for episodic therapy of recurrent genital herpes are shown in Table 9.2 below.

As you can see from the discussion above, antiviral therapy used for recurrent genital herpes gives less dramatic results than it does in first episodes. This is partly explained by the fact that the immune system is doing a lot of the work already. That's why recurrent outbreaks are usually much shorter than first episodes, anyway. Many people feel the additional gains from episodic ther-

TABLE 9.2. Recommended oral antiviral regimens for episodic therapy of recurrent genital herpes*

Name	Brand	Regimen*
Acyclovir	(generic)	200 mg, 5 times daily for 5 days*
Acyclovir	(generic)	400 mg, 3 times daily for 5 days*
Acyclovir	(generic)	800 mg, 2 times daily for 5 days*
Famciclovir	Famvir®	125 mg, 2 times daily for 5 days*
Valacyclovir	Valtrex®	500 mg, 2 times daily for 3 days*
Valacyclovir	Valtrex®	500 mg, 2 times daily for 5 days*

*Episodic therapy should be initiated at the onset of prodromal symptoms (or at first sign of infection if no prodrome is detected).

apy are marginal, but for others, medication offers a useful way to manage outbreaks. This is especially true for the person whose outbreaks tend to last more than a week.

Episodic therapy has its best results when medication is begun at the first sign of prodrome. For this reason, those taking episodic therapy should keep a supply of medication on hand so that they can start treatment when they first notice prodromal symptoms. The time required to involve a healthcare provider in this decision and obtain medication causes a significant delay in the start of treatment and is impractical. Most healthcare providers, therefore, will be open to this arrangement. If recurrent lesions are already present, on the other hand, therapy usually offers little benefit.

SUPPRESSIVE THERAPY — People with herpes who want to eliminate (suppress) outbreaks altogether can take antiviral medication daily to hold HSV in check. Suppressive therapy reduces the number of outbreaks by at least 75% among people with frequent recurrences (that is, six or more outbreaks a year). For some people, suppressive therapy can prevent outbreaks altogether. Recommended antiviral dosages for the suppression of recurrent genital herpes are shown in Table 9.3 below.

As in the case of Teri, at the start of this chapter, many people find that suppressive antiviral treatment radically changes their experience of herpes, especially if they have frequent outbreaks. A long-term study has enrolled people who had frequent recurrences, put them on an acyclovir dose of 400 mg twice daily, and carefully tracked the results. In publishing the five-year data, researchers reported that nearly all patients on suppressive therapy had a dramatic reduction in the number of their outbreaks, beginning in the first year. They also found that people on this regimen experienced fewer and fewer recurrences, so that after one

TABLE 9.3. Recommended oral antiviral regimens for suppression of recurrent genital herpes

Name	Brand	Regimen
Acyclovir	(generic)	400 mg, 2 times daily every day
Famciclovir	Famvir®	250 mg, 2 times daily every day
Valacyclovir	Valtrex®	500 mg, once daily every day—*for people with fewer than 10 outbreaks per year*
Valacyclovir	Valtrex®	1000 mg, once daily every day, or 500 mg, twice daily—*for people with 10 or more outbreaks per year*

year, more than half of patients on suppressive therapy were completely free of outbreaks. A total of 20% of study participants had no outbreaks for the entire five years of the study. In a follow-up report on the patients in the 5-year study, 239 patients stopped acyclovir suppressive therapy after 6 years of successful suppression: 86% had at least one recurrence within a median of 68 days of stopping suppressive therapy and 75% had at least two recurrences within a median of 180 days after stopping suppressive therapy. Famciclovir and valacyclovir, both approved in 1995, have fewer years of history behind them, but one-year studies have shown that both drugs give similarly dramatic reductions in the number of outbreaks for most people.

In addition to the reduction in symptoms, suppressive antiviral therapy also has been studied for its potential benefits in improving patients' psychological and social adjustment. A recent multinational study found that suppressive therapy was correlated with statistically significant improvement in quality of life after 6 and 12 months of treatment.

While suppressive therapy can be remarkably successful, it's important to note that some individuals simply do not respond this well to a particular antiviral medication. In some cases, an increased dose is required to suppress HSV or a different medication is worth trying. For example, those who do not respond well to acyclovir may need as much as 800 mg twice daily or may do better on one of the prodrugs. In a smaller number of cases, antivirals simply are not effective, suggesting the need for a different approach.

On the other end of the spectrum, people sometimes experiment with taking a smaller dose of antivirals, reporting that they need only 400 mg per day of acyclovir instead of the usual 800 mg, for example. Various regimens have been studied, and from the published research it seems that in general the effectiveness of suppressive therapy increases with the frequency of dosing. If you're wanting to alter the recommended suppressive therapy regimen, it's a good idea to discuss the issue with your medical professional.

Those on suppressive therapy may wish to stay on the drug indefinitely, and in the case of acyclovir, the safety of continuous therapy is established for up to 9 years. But many experts in the field argue that most patients should talk with their healthcare providers about possibly discontinuing suppressive treatment after 12 consecutive months for what amounts to a reality check—to see if the need persists. Sometimes they won't have any outbreaks even without the drug, probably because of HSV's tendency to become less active after a number of years. Some people also find that their recurrences are less bothersome, so that they no longer want to take daily medication. The problem is that you have no way of knowing unless treatment is stopped for a while. For patients who continue to have a need for therapy, it can be renewed.

SAFETY CONCERNS

Over the years, many people with herpes have written ASHA with questions about the long-term safety of antiviral medication, particularly as used in suppressive therapy. Do these drugs have any toxic effects? Is suppressive therapy likely to give rise to drug-resistant strains of the virus or to weaken the body's natural immune response?

Suppressive therapy with acyclovir has been studied in thousands of patients over the past 15 years, and so far it appears to be very safe. In large trials, a small number of patients report side effects such as headaches, nausea, or diarrhea, but overall these complaints are rare. Researchers also have run laboratory tests to check for systemic effects of the drug on liver function, white blood cell count, and various other indexes of good health. So far, there is no evidence acyclovir causes harm to any internal organs. It will be years before researchers have gathered as much data on valacyclovir and famciclovir as they have now on acyclovir. However, thus far the safety data on the newer drugs are comparable to those for acyclovir.

The issue of resistant strains is more complicated. Within the universe of HSV-2, there are many different *strains* of the virus. For the most part, the differences among them are relevant only to molecular biologists. A small number of strains, however, are less sensitive to the effects of the three antiviral drugs that we have discussed in this chapter. One reason for this lack of sensitivity is that some strains actually lack the enzyme (thymidine kinase) that triggers these drugs and enables them to thwart the virus in its effort to spread. These strains are rare, can arise spontaneously, and typically have only a small proportion of viral particles that lack thymidine kinase. For this reason, the immune system generally can control these viral strains in healthy people.

In patients who have weakened immune systems, however, these strains can cause serious illness, because the immune system can't do its customary work in suppressing herpes, and resistant strains can replicate without much interference. People with

AIDS, for example, may have severe herpes outbreaks that do not heal with conventional antiviral medication. Alternate treatments are now being used for these patients.

Is the problem of drug resistance likely to increase over time, as more and more people take antivirals? This is a controversial issue, but it appears unlikely. On one hand, researchers have actually checked samples of HSV taken before the development of acyclovir, and they find a small percentage of viral strains that are naturally less sensitive to the drug. Given this finding, resistance would appear to be more a matter of chance or of immune deficiency than the result of acyclovir use. On the other hand, some scientists believe that HSV does mutate over time, and it's possible that acyclovir—or any antiviral drug—will exert pressure for certain strains of the virus to survive better than others.

For now, the experts say, the odds of developing acyclovir-resistant herpes are extremely low in people with normal immune systems. Researchers have looked for resistant strains in people taking acyclovir daily for up to 6 years and found no evidence of increasing resistance. A recent survey of herpes patients in northwest England reported that resistant strains of the herpes virus were found with equal prevalence (0.1% to 0.6% of virus samples tested) among immunocompetent patients who had been treated with acyclovir and among those who had not received acyclovir. The issue of drug-resistance in those with weakened immunity, by contrast, is of more immediate concern, and immunocompromised patients with herpes should be monitored closely if they're taking antiviral medication.

ANTIVIRALS AND
SUBCLINICAL SHEDDING

While antivirals can be successful in controlling herpes symptoms, researchers only recently have turned their attention to the important issue of antiviral therapy and asymptomatic shedding. Does suppressive therapy lower the risk of unrecognized herpes reactivation as well as curb recognized outbreaks? Does it change the odds of spreading herpes to a sexual partner?

One study addressing this question found that women on suppressive acyclovir (400 mg, twice daily) had a 94% reduction in subclinical shedding while taking daily therapy. This type of study has also been done with famciclovir and valacyclovir, yielding similar reductions in both men and women. Given that antivirals can reduce viral shedding both with symptoms and without, it's logical to suppose that treatment has an impact on transmission. The researchers who conducted these studies, however, caution that even daily therapy did not totally block viral shedding in all patients, and the amounts of virus found on some days of shedding were probably sufficient to cause transmission. Because of its obvious importance to people with herpes, the role of therapy as a means of preventing the spread of the infection is being examined closely. A study of whether suppressive valacyclovir can help prevent transmission is expected to report its results by 2002.

COMPARISON SHOPPING

How does one evaluate the available treatments? Let's consider four major aspects: effectiveness, safety, convenience, and cost.

In terms of effectiveness, clinical studies have not found any significant differences among acyclovir, famciclovir, and valacyclovir in terms of their effectiveness for people with established HSV infection. All three appear to work for the vast majority of patients as a suppressive therapy and to have modest but predictable benefit as episodic therapy.

As for safety, it can be argued that acyclovir has an edge by virtue of its long track record, with no evidence of toxicity even in those who have been taking daily medication for years. However, the newer drugs also appear to be very safe and have few side effects. Valacyclovir, which uses acyclovir as its active ingredient, has shown a similar safety profile so far, as has famciclovir. Perhaps, with time, the prodrugs will match acyclovir's record fully.

Convenience probably offers an edge to the newer drugs. Valacyclovir and famciclovir can be taken twice daily as episodic therapies for recurrent herpes, compared with three to five times daily for acyclovir. For suppression, valacyclovir achieves good results in most people with a once-daily dose, something that neither of its competitors has been able to match.

Cost, of course, is the other critical variable. Here there is actually good news. In the seven years since this book was first published, the availability of generic acyclovir, price competition among national chain pharmacies, the advent of on-line pharmacies, and increased utilization of prescription drug cards by insurers have combined to make antiviral medication more affordable and easier to obtain. Nonetheless, in today's healthcare arena, a given patient's therapeutic options are highly dependent on the insurer's regulations and policies. One type of health plan might place generic acyclovir in its formulary; another might go with one of the prodrugs.

If, on the other hand, you will be paying out of pocket for a long-term course of therapy, it would be smart to research the cost of each of the three drugs to determine which is the best value in your particular market. For suppressive therapy, for example, what is the cost to you of twice daily generic acyclovir versus once daily valacyclovir? How does your local pharmacy's price compare with those of the national chains? And what are the on-line pharmacies charging? A recent survey by ASHA showed an enormous range in prices for six months of suppressive therapy though on-line vendors. Prices were as low as $150 for six months of suppressive therapy with generic drug supplied by an on-line pharmacy, and discounts could be found for the prodrugs as well.

In the end, all three antivirals can be considered safe and effective, but the hit to one's pocketbook may vary dramatically according to health insurance, geography, and the pricing structure at your preferred pharmacy.

OTHER ANTIVIRAL DRUGS

Foscarnet is used as an alternative therapy for immunocompromised patients who don't respond well to acyclovir. Like acyclovir, foscarnet blocks viral replication, but it does so by working directly against a viral enzyme called *polymerase*. The drug has been helpful, particularly to people with AIDS, but it has several disadvantages. First, it isn't readily absorbed through the stomach, and must be administered intravenously. Second, it has many toxic side effects. Foscarnet is not currently recommended for patients with normal immune function. Another antiviral compound, *trifluridine*, is occasionally used to treat herpes infections that do not heal on acyclovir. A number of other antivirals fall into the category of topical or investigational drugs.

TOPICAL THERAPY

The most effective form of therapy for HSV infection is oral antiviral therapy, but because herpes was originally perceived as a skin condition, the idea of topical medication has always had some appeal. Over the past three decades a number of different compounds have been developed for topical application to herpes lesions, though it has proved difficult to make a drug that's absorbed through the skin well enough to provide substantial relief. Acyclovir was initially tested and approved as a topical ointment for genital herpes in 1982. Results with oral acyclovir were far superior, however, and since 1985, acyclovir cream has not been recommended for genital herpes. Although none of the topical therapies studied so far has been on par with oral therapy, the effort to develop more effective topicals continues.

PENCICLOVIR — Penciclovir is available as a topical cream and has been investigated for the treatment of oral and genital herpes. A 1% penciclovir cream known as Denavir® can be purchased over the counter for treatment of cold sores on the lips and face. This topical formulation shortens the duration of pain and healing time for cold sore patients when applied every two hours (during waking hours) and also appears to reduce viral shedding. The usefulness of this drug for genital herpes, however, remains questionable. A randomized, double-blind comparison of penciclovir cream and acyclovir cream for genital herpes found no clinically significant differences between the two drugs. Acyclovir cream is no longer recommended for genital herpes because oral therapy is much more effective.

DOCOSANOL — Recently, the U. S. Food & Drug Administration approved a new nonprescription cream medication for oral herpes—*docosanol*. Docosanol's mode of action is different from that of acyclovir or penciclovir; docosanol is thought to disrupt the process by which the herpes virus particle gains entry to the uninfected cell. One small placebo-controlled study (63 patients) of docosanol for recurrent cold sores found that early application, i.e., at first "tingling sensation" or at the first appearance of any redness, shortened healing time by approximately 3 days. This product has not been studied thoroughly for genital herpes.

OTHER INVESTIGATIONAL DRUGS — One of the most promising topical treatments for genital herpes in recent years is a compound known as resiquimod, originally developed by 3M Pharmaceuticals and now licensed to Eli Lilly and Company. Resiquimod belongs to a new class of drug called immune modulators, and its developers are conducting Phase III clinical trials (see Chapter 17).

A topical gel, cidofovir (sometimes designated *SP-303*), has been used experimentally, with some success, to treat herpes infection in AIDS patients. In a placebo-controlled study in non-

AIDS patients with recent onset of a recurrence of anogenital herpes, cidofovir gel shortened the duration of viral shedding at lesion sites but had no significant effect on lesion healing time.

Several other topical drugs and organic compounds with therapeutic potential for oral herpes have been studied clinically, including balm mint extract; undecyclenic acid (the active anti-fungal ingredient in Desenex®); ascorbic acid solution; and 3% foscarnet cream. One controlled study in genital herpes patients compared acyclovir cream with a topical ointment containing Canadian propolis and reported faster healing and resolution of symptoms with propolis, but we mention here again that acyclovir cream is no longer recommended for genital herpes because the oral form of the drug gives substantially better results. None of these investigational substances is currently approved for the treatment of oral or genital herpes.

TOPICAL ANESTHETICS — Other topical drugs, while they make no claim to stop viral replication, may relieve symptoms in other ways. Topical lidocaine partially (and temporarily) numbs the nerve endings and is occasionally used to treat the pain of first episodes. However, it's not widely used for herpes, and people using it should be aware of the possibility of allergic reactions to this and similar drugs such as novocaine. The FDA recently approved a patch version of topical lidocaine (Lidoderm®) for the symptomatic treatment of post-herpetic neuralgia, the very painful after-effect of the herpes zoster viral infection known as *shingles*, though the usefulness of this for HSV-related neuralgia has not been studied. A recent placebo-controlled study of 1.8% tetracaine cream for oral herpes reported a 30% reduction in healing time (about 2 days); patients also reported meaningful improvement in lesion-related itching.

OTC MEDICATIONS — Most of the medications used for genital herpes are discussed in the previous sections on antivirals, but there are a few others worth noting. In particular, people with herpes sometimes try over-the-counter products to relieve the symptoms of a flare-up. It's difficult to assess the value of these medications because they generally are not tested as rigorously as the other drugs discussed in this chapter and are not evaluated in the scientific literature. In some cases, neither are they labeled specifically for use in the treatment of genital herpes. They nonetheless attract attention through word-of-mouth, or because they claim to erase whatever kind of symptom is most distressing to the patient—itching, for example.

Unfortunately, topical creams may actually delay the healing of herpes outbreaks. In some cases, the creams contain alcohol compounds that might dry the skin to the point where it is easily chafed. Other topical treatments, such as Campho-Phenique®, may make patients feel better because the product contains phenol. Like xylocaine and lidocaine, phenol numbs the area locally, without treating the actual infection. Some people may find this useful. It's important to note, however, that products such as Campho-Phenique® or Blistex® do not actually work directly against the virus—they concentrate instead on the symptoms of viral attack.

Other topical medications—even prescription drugs—can have a down side when it comes to herpes. Some doctors use topical steroid creams to reduce inflammation and speed healing for a variety of skin problems. Unfortunately, steroids cause some immune impairment, and this may make a herpesvirus infection worse, decreasing the ability of the skin to heal on its own. Steroids are not effective for HSV, and they can prolong herpes outbreaks. Topical steroids such as hydrocortisone may increase the risk of yeast infection as well. (By the way, people taking steroids for other conditions, such as asthma, sometimes report that their herpes outbreaks are worse as a result.)

If you want more information about a prescription or over-the-counter product for treating symptoms of genital herpes, one option is to contact the Office of Consumer Affairs at the FDA. (See the Resource List on page 221.) They can discuss drugs that are labeled specifically for treatment of genital herpes. Another option is to contact the product's manufacturer.

ALTERNATIVE THERAPIES

Among those who find herpes troubling, some look for alternatives in managing the infection, often because of the expense or the inconvenience of prescription medications, or because they have philosophical objections to them. They look for other ways to take control. In ASHA's 1991 survey, most patients had tried from two to five different therapies for genital herpes. Some of these were not strictly drugs but dietary supplements or nutritional approaches. Some were various types of stress reduction or psychotherapy. There are advocates for hypnosis, homeopathy, acupuncture, naturopathy, chiropractic, psychotherapy, visualization, group therapy, dietary changes, herbal remedies, 12-step groups, traditional Chinese medicine, and more. The list is long, and it grows each year. The movement toward alternative medicine, in fact, is a national trend of considerable scope. According to a survey published in 1998, more than 42% of Americans were using an alternative therapy in 1997—up from 33% in 1990. It's estimated that we spend $27 billion a year in the process. Partly as a result, the National Institutes of Health has now set up a special branch, the Center for Alternative and Complementary Medicine.

Unfortunately, until some of these studies in alternative medicine are completed and published, it's difficult to evaluate alternative therapies for herpes. The fact is that most are not scientifically tested and retested like prescription drugs. In the vast majority of cases, there are no double-blind studies, so one can never be sure that the results would have appeared the same to an unconvinced observer. These therapies also lack an approval process that hinges on the performance of a given treatment in a large cross-section of people. What we're left with in most cases are the personal accounts of a few individuals who have tried something, found it successful for them, and either want to share what they've learned or find out whether the approach is medically safe.

Because ASHA is asked about many of these treatments, we wish we were in a better position to broker solid information. Sadly, we don't have much hard evidence about many of the alternative therapies suggested. We can, however, share what we know about the approaches most commonly used by people with recurrent genital herpes.

VITAMINS, MINERALS, AMINO ACIDS — These days, it seems, nutrition gets the credit or the blame for a host of physical and mental ailments. And you can include herpes on the list. Some people praise the benefits of removing coffee, alcohol, or yeast from their diet, saying that this reduces the frequency of outbreaks. Others suggest supplementing the diet with substances such as the mineral zinc or vitamins C and E.

Perhaps the most often tried nutritional approach is use of the dietary supplement L-lysine. One of the essential amino acids that the body uses to build proteins, L-lysine is a natural part of many foods we consume, such as meat, milk, and eggs. Beginning in the late 1970s, a small number of nutritional researchers began to claim that people who consumed abnormally large quantities of lysine on a daily basis had fewer herpes flare-ups and recovered from them more quickly. In one study, subjects took 3,000 mg of lysine every day to achieve these gains. Unfortunately, other studies found that lysine was ineffective.

While interest in lysine therapy seems to have waned over the past decade, it still has a fairly strong word-of-mouth approval in some circles. Typical is this letter from Preston: "I started taking lysine every day, but I wasn't consistent. I would run out, then get more pills in a month or two. Then I started taking 500 mg every single day, and I haven't had an outbreak in a year. I don't care if it's all in my mind, as long as I get results."

The consensus in the scientific community is that lysine supplements in particular have no inherent value. Experts also say that if you feel your diet is deficient in some way and you want to take a supplement, the best bet is a broad-spectrum, multivitamin formula that meets the Recommended Daily Allowance (RDA) for the nutrients listed. According to many experts in the field, nutrition is a complex *interaction* of various elements, and people are best served by eating a balanced diet that gives them all the essential nutrients from real food. (We do need lysine, and a balanced diet probably contains something on the order of 500 mg a day.) On the other hand, *megadoses* of any one amino acid or vitamin can easily throw the body's chemical system out of balance.

At one time, advocates of lysine also suggested *restricting* dietary intake of another amino acid, arginine, which is found in lots of common foods, among them chocolate, nuts, corn, and beer. Some people have found that, for them, arginine-rich foods seem to trigger outbreaks. Nutritional research in recent years, however, shows that arginine actually enhances immune function and helps people resist some infections. It's been tested on burn patients, for example, and has been shown to lower rates of secondary infection.

If all this seems confusing and contradictory to you, you're not alone. The one area of general agreement seems to be this: If your diet is inadequate in some way, this can definitely have a negative effect on your health and your resistance to infections. Seeking help from a nutritionist may be a good idea. He or she probably will not be able to control herpes specifically with dietary changes, but the benefits to your health as a whole may carry over to herpes.

OTHER REMEDIES — Beyond the vitamins, minerals, and amino acids of a balanced diet, there remains a good deal of interest in specific remedies. Goldenseal, for example, is an herb that is thought to have antiviral properties, and some people use it for herpes, either in capsules or strong teas. Garlic, an ancient folk remedy for colds, has been shown to inhibit a number of viruses and bacteria in the laboratory, herpes among them. Some people, therefore, take garlic in capsules, and they report good results. Practitioners of homeopathic medicine, naturopathic medicine, and Chinese herbal medicine also have treatments for people with herpes. We wish we could say more about these approaches, but they simply haven't been rigorously tested for their effects on HSV in large numbers of people.

There also can be health risks associated with nonconventional herpes remedies. Some people, for example, have used dye-light therapy for herpes, a practice that can cause cancerous changes in healthy cells. And many topical creams or oils— including over-the-counter products such as cortisone creams— will actually slow the healing of herpes lesions.

It's also worth considering that some alternative therapies, even megadoses of vitamins, are quite costly. If you have frequent outbreaks, antiviral therapy may give you significantly more benefit for your drugstore dollar than nutritional supplements or herbal remedies.

Learning more about the pros and cons of alternative therapies is not easy, but the coming years should bring us more information about the safety and effectiveness of various approaches.

THE "HEALTHY LIFESTYLE" — Each of us might have a different definition of the healthy lifestyle, but there seems to be broad agreement that, regardless of herpes, certain behaviors help keep us operating at peak performance. These include eating a balanced diet, getting the proper amount of sleep and exercise, avoiding excesses of caffeine and alcohol, staying away from tobacco, and being careful to manage chronic stress. Medical science has had a lot to say about the benefits of these "lifestyle choices" as they apply to cancer, heart disease, and various other important health problems.

Many sing the praises of the healthy lifestyle when it comes to herpes, as well. "Herpes has really forced me to look at my life and set priorities," says one woman. "Now I watch what I eat, get plenty of sleep, and have become an avid jogger. I feel so much better, and my outbreaks seem to be less and less a problem."

As in the case of alternative medicines, the comments generally are not based on rigorous science. But the basic health lessons of childhood—beginning with "eat your vegetables"—seem to hold merit for lots of people.

In a way, you might regard herpes as you would the common cold. You know that your body is constantly challenged by various germs. But even when there is a cold "going around" your family or your office, your immune system often protects you. Then, if you lose sleep or just get generally "run down," suddenly you've lost the battle and you've got that cold. The object of the healthy lifestyle is precisely this: Don't run that body down.

CONSIDERING TREATMENT FOR YOURSELF

In today's healthcare environment, a person diagnosed with first episode genital herpes is most likely to receive a course of antiviral therapy to eliminate these initial symptoms. But what then? Is it best to keep a supply of an antiviral on hand in case of recurrences? Is daily suppressive therapy something to consider? Who makes the call?

There are no simple guidelines to offer, because every patient's circumstances are different. The patient's medical history, the impact of herpes on the patient's life, and the patient's and healthcare provider's views regarding treatment—all come into play.

Ideally, however, one constant here will be a dialogue between patient and provider concerning the impact of herpes and the therapeutic options. Here are some issues to weigh:

- What is the infecting type: HSV-1 or HSV-2? As we explained earlier, HSV-1 is unlikely to cause a pattern of frequent recurrences and appears less likely to cause asymptomatic shedding as well. With HSV-2, on the other hand, symptomatic recurrences are virtually a sure thing, and rates of asymptomatic shedding are higher.

- Are you already experiencing a pattern of frequent or painful outbreaks? A pattern of recurrent outbreaks six or more times a year leads some patients to use suppressive antiviral therapy, especially if the outbreaks are lengthy or painful. But the threshold is different for everyone. In any case, your doctor has no way to gauge this other than your honest assessment. Try to communicate this information.

- Is anxiety about recurrences substantially affecting your life? Does recurrent herpes take an emotional toll on you? Even people who get just a handful of outbreaks each year may feel the need for therapy if, for example, they are facing a time of stress during which herpes is the last thing they want to contend with. One example: Persons recently divorced or on their own after the breakup of a long-term relationship might suddenly feel anxiety about herpes and seek advice on treatment for the first time.

• Do your recurrences last a long time? The average duration of recurrences is about five to seven days, and in these cases, episodic treatment may not bring a substantial improvement. Persons with longer recurrences might benefit significantly from episodic treatments. Those with frequent but brief recurrences might get more benefit from suppressive treatment.

• Are you pregnant, or trying to get pregnant? Most of the medications mentioned here should not be used during pregnancy, except in very specific circumstances. (See Chapter 14 for more on herpes in pregnancy.)

• Are you and your partner very concerned about the risk of transmission? The usefulness of antiviral medication in helping prevent transmission has not been proven, but for people who want to do everything they can to reduce the risk, suppressive therapy can be a reasonable addition to other prevention strategies.

Once they have gone through a first episode and have learned more about genital herpes, some people may feel no need to use antiviral therapy. Others, however, may be helped by a regimen of suppressive therapy or by a refillable prescription for treating recurrences.

Among healthcare professionals, the standard approach has been to watch and wait as a newly diagnosed patient establishes a pattern of recurrences and then prescribe accordingly. Suppressive therapy, traditionally, would be reserved for patients with frequent or troublesome recurrences. However, based on studies showing that suppressive therapy also may improve quality of life, some physicians have adopted a more liberal approach. Studies are now under way to evaluate the idea of routinely treating HSV-2 patients with suppressive therapy in the first six months following diagnosis, on the theory that this will aid in the psychosocial adjustment process.

The most important piece of advice here is to focus on your needs and speak up for yourself in this decision-making process. All too often, patients receive a prescription for treatment of a first episode and then get little followup in the next few months. If a patient is somewhat embarrassed to bring up the subject, the result is that they have little or no chance to discuss the impact of herpes and the potential role of treatment.

10

SORTING OUT THE EMOTIONAL ISSUES

〜

"When I acquired herpes seven months ago," says Sean, "I was shattered. I remember sitting there in the dark listening to Pink Floyd's 'Comfortably Numb,' which is exactly what I was (thanks to the sedatives my doctor had given me)."

When we're first diagnosed with genital herpes, much of what we learn has to do with the physical impact of herpes: the types of symptoms, the pattern of outbreaks, or factors that may trigger outbreaks. But it's well-accepted by now that for many people herpes also has emotional consequences. There are dozens of behavioral studies that have assessed the social and psychological effects of herpes. Especially in the first few weeks and months, herpes can affect self-image, make one feel isolated or embarrassed, and complicate relationships. For some of us, these issues can be just as troublesome—and sometimes much more so—than its physical symptoms.

The good news is that these problems tend to fade away with time. In fact, some studies show that even six months can make a big difference in adjusting to herpes.

Your own response depends on the circumstances of your

life. For some, the emotional impact of herpes may be minimal, even at the start. If, however, there are some tough personal issues raised by a recent herpes diagnosis, it can be very helpful to sort them out, analyze what's upsetting you, and think through some approaches to resolving them.

HERPES AND SELF-IMAGE

Many people describe herpes as shaking their self-confidence or making them think themselves less worthy. For example, a young woman who had acquired herpes as a teenager wrote: "I had times when I would feel very unattractive and feel like I was different from everyone my own age. The best way I can sum it up is that I felt 'dirty.'"

Why does herpes have the power to alter our self-image? In some ways this is truly a paradox. HSV is a common virus, and most adults already have HSV-1, the usual cause of cold sores. Most of us have had other herpesviruses as well. Examples include the viruses that cause chickenpox, mononucleosis, and the childhood infection roseola.

Psychologists point out that numerous chronic health conditions adversely affect self-image or self-esteem, and this seems to be an issue with herpes. The lack of a cure and the prospect of recurrent symptoms are stressful thoughts for some as they think through what herpes will mean for their lives.

Too often we see health as an all-or-nothing proposition—we are either healthy or unhealthy, with no middle ground. And some people regard a chronic infection like herpes as the end of health. We become somehow imperfect.

In reality, however, health involves a process of growth and change. Everyone faces a host of physical challenges as inevitable as life itself. Whether it's a cold, the flu, allergies, an ear infection, or anything else, the task is to meet them head on and get past them. Herpes is no exception. In the end, we should consider ourselves healthy because we meet the challenges that life throws our way.

Herpes can also threaten our self-image in an area where many of us feel a bit vulnerable already: our feelings of sexual desirability. Sociologist Sevgi Aral comments that people carry around with them a good deal of general anxiety about their attractiveness to a potential partner. Feelings of insecurity such as these are commonplace, and herpes adds a complication.

The impact of herpes on one's sex life might be challenging, but this too can be addressed—first, by learning to talk about it, and second, by making rational decisions about protecting a partner. Studies show that, with time, newly diagnosed persons usually overcome the distress they often feel about the effect of herpes on sexual relationships. We will discuss this further in Chapter 12.

SOCIAL STIGMA?

Closely connected to the issue of self-image is the matter of how we believe others see us. In many cases, the person with herpes will assume that society regards him or her as different in some substantial way. This, in essence, is the definition of social stigma. It's a feeling that one is *marked* by herpes—that it's more just than a medical condition.

Part of the reason that a mundane illness like herpes causes problems—even temporarily—is that we fear what others may think about us.

Interestingly, though, sociologists who study this topic point out that people may assume that something carries social stigma when it doesn't, or may exaggerate the potential for stigma. A joke you remember from years ago, a less-than-sensitive remark by a doctor—these sorts of experiences can cast a long shadow psychologically. On the other hand, talking to a close friend about herpes may show you an entirely different reality. Lots of people know that herpes is a very common infection, and lots of people know someone who has herpes.

So why don't they talk about it more? One reason that herpes raises issues of social stigma is the fact that, as a society, we're just beginning to feel more comfortable talking about sex and sexuality in general. Today, we're surrounded by the imagery of sex in arts, entertainment, and advertising of products as diverse as soft drinks and automobiles. There are some signs as well that on a personal level we are becoming somewhat more open about sexuality—more likely to discuss topics such as sexual orientation and sexual function. All the same, these topics still are not the easiest things in the world to bring up in conversation. A good example is the enormous amount of press and conversation triggered by the launch of Viagra in 1998, including the television commercials featuring retired U.S. Senator Bob Dole. As a society we certainly talked about the issue of sexual dysfunction as we never had before, but we still had some discomfort and embarrassment with something that had long been kept out of public discourse. Hence the spate of jokes and editorial cartoons.

With herpes, there is a similar trend to more awareness and openness. Prime-time television advertising appears to have raised awareness, and surveys show that the public is much better educated about the subject today than ever before. Perhaps the day will come when even the idea of social stigma connected to herpes is a distant memory.

TALKING ABOUT HERPES

In the meantime, of course, it may be a bit awkward or embarrassing to discuss herpes with various people in your life, and many people worry for a while about the practical impact of herpes on important relationships. Do you dare tell people? Will discussing herpes damage a relationship you have now? Will a future romantic interest understand and accept the news?

These anxieties are natural, but it's important to overcome them. If you are withdrawing from friends or intimate relationships because of what you've internalized as social stigma, you run the risk of cutting yourself off from the support you need to keep everything in perspective. Studies have shown that social support is one of the most important factors in ensuring that herpes doesn't interfere with your life over the long haul.

Psychologist Cal VanderPlate, who has studied the behavioral effects of herpes, says that the key to keeping herpes in perspective is communication. People who can tell a partner or a friend about herpes often get emotional support from this person when they need it.

Talking about herpes, even with someone you love and trust, can be daunting at first. And herpes isn't likely to be something that you will choose to bring up with just anyone. In surveys, people most frequently report discussing herpes with their healthcare provider and with their spouse or partner, though not everyone does.

Perhaps the most pressing worry for those newly diagnosed with herpes is the reaction of a sexual partner. Feelings of suspicion or resentment can be a factor in some cases, as a couple tries to sort out the source of the herpes infection. On the other hand, if blame is not an issue, those who already have a steady partner potentially have a wonderful source of emotional support that can ease their adjustment to herpes.

People often say they especially fear telling a *new* partner or romantic interest because they're afraid of being rejected. They particularly worry about herpes being contagious, and about how the conversation is going to go when they have to talk about which precautions they might use. "I've had herpes for three months now, and I've been avoiding any sexual entanglements," writes Pat. "I'm not ready to tell anyone. I just don't think I'll be able to handle it if someone rejects me because of this." Experts say the best way to approach talking to a partner about herpes is to think through what you are going to say—perhaps even rehearse it—and then say it in a direct, honest, and upbeat way. (Telling a partner and thinking through the issue of prevention are explored in depth in the next two chapters.)

Support can come from a friend as well. In any case, the key is having someone to talk to, but this requires honesty and openness on the part of the person with herpes. Usually, says VanderPlate, acceptance and support are just around the corner, but we never know unless we take the risk. You may need a little time first, but opening up to a trusted friend may be exactly the boost you need to put things in perspective and get on with your life.

HERPES AND SEXUAL HEALTH

As we mentioned earlier, sexuality appears to be an area where most people experience insecurity from time to time, and having a chronic infection that is sexually transmitted can exacerbate these insecurities. In addition, there are practical issues. Having an infection that can reactivate and become contagious at unpredictable times does present some challenges. Herpes can interfere with sex when symptoms are present. And it can raise the issue of condom use or other risk reduction measures between outbreaks.

As with other aspects of the emotional and social adjustment to having herpes, surveys show that some people find herpes affects their enjoyment of sex and their spontaneity. But here again, the negative effects are often short-term. After a period of adjustment, most people have sex just as often and enjoy it just as much as they did before.

Most people with herpes naturally do worry about transmitting herpes to a sexual partner, and having a sexual relationship does mean considering the risks: When is herpes active? What, precisely, are *my* symptoms? Is my partner at risk—or does he or she already have it? Do we need to use condoms or some other form of risk reduction?

There *are* things you can do to lower the risk of spreading herpes. Experts believe that simply knowing your symptoms and refraining from sexual contact during symptomatic times is an important precaution. Use of condoms in between outbreaks also has value in lowering risks. And it's known that medication may be helpful in reducing the number of days during which the virus is active and *shedding* on the surface of your skin. All of these issues are covered in more detail in Chapter 12.

In addition to the sexual impact of herpes, people often wonder if the burden of having herpes—and possibly transmitting it—will become a serious problem over the long term. ASHA has interviewed many couples about this issue and found no indication that herpes has to stand in the way of successful, enduring relationships. One woman who doesn't have herpes wrote ASHA with the specific aim of making this very point. "Some people with herpes seem to give up on relationships," she commented, "so I wanted to share my story. My husband is the love of my life. We've been married almost 10 years, and herpes hasn't spoiled our relationship in any way. Like almost everyone else, we've had our problems, but herpes isn't one of them."

Asked about herpes and long-term relationships, psychologists concur that it's basically a non-issue in a healthy relationship. As long as two people are honest with each other at the start, as long as they can talk about herpes and make choices about it, the infection itself becomes just one more practical matter to deal with—usually a small one. If herpes triggers a lot of tension in a relationship, the experts say, often there are some underlying problems.

EMOTIONS AND ADJUSTMENT

Issues of self-esteem, fear of rejection, and anxieties about one's sex life are common among those newly diagnosed, and herpes can have other emotional consequences as well. A number of studies have documented generalized anxiety in a percentage of newly diagnosed patients as well as feelings of depression or other signs of psychological distress. As we have mentioned earlier, however, even those who have initially had a difficult time with herpes often go through a process of adjustment after which they are functioning—and feeling—much the way they had before their diagnosis.

In ASHA's 1991 survey, signs of emotional stress were quite common during the period following a first episode. These included feelings of depression, noted by 82% of respondents, fear of rejection (75%), feelings of isolation (69%), fear of discovery (55%), and self-destructive feelings (27%).

Many of those surveyed, however, had been coping with herpes for several years. Interestingly, when they were asked about the most recent 12 months (prior to the survey), the results were markedly different: Fewer people had the same fears and feelings.

In raising the possibility of consequences such as depression, our purpose is not to characterize herpes as psychologically crippling. Rather it's to allow for the possibility that a newly diagnosed patient may have a wide variety of emotional responses. Though these responses are usually short-term, a person who is suffering greatly may benefit from taking aggressive steps to treat herpes and to seek help from a professional counselor who can help sort through the issues that the diagnosis has raised.

MOVING FORWARD

If having herpes is causing you a lot of emotional stress, here are some points to keep in mind:

• Realize that it's normal to be stressed emotionally by herpes, especially at first. Give yourself some time to adjust, and remember that the emotional issues will get easier.

• Keep in mind that genital herpes is somewhat like other infections you may have had in the past. You are capable of managing it.

• If you're feeling isolated, you may need to find someone to talk to. Perhaps you might pick one close friend and tell her or him about it. You can ask that the conversation be kept in absolute confidence.

• Try not to make the assumption that having herpes will prevent you from being romantically involved or having successful long-term relationships. There are millions of couples in which one or both partners have this infection. For the vast majority, the relationships stand or fall on far more important issues.

11

TELLING A PARTNER

⟨◎⟩

Carl, now 38, remembers the first few conversations he had about herpes. "When I got the diagnosis, I was able to make phone calls to the two people I'd been intimate with and ask if either of them had any idea they had herpes. I wasn't so much angry at that point as worried and wanting to be, I guess, responsible about it. So it wasn't that hard to make the calls. But later, when it came time to tell someone new, I lost my nerve at first. I really couldn't stand the idea that it might make someone feel differently about me."

The prospect of telling another person you have herpes can make you anxious, especially when you're getting ready to tell someone with whom you'd like to be sexually intimate. What will this person say? Laugh? Cry? Accept that herpes doesn't have to be a big deal?

It's an important conversation—one that can break the ice and set the relationship on a very positive course. Its outcome is not completely in your control. But there are things you can do to shape the message and the response.

MAKING THE CHOICE

As some people ponder having this kind of "heart-to-heart" with a lover or romantic interest, they begin to wonder if it's really necessary. Why risk rejection, they reason, when there may be another way? What about just avoiding sex during herpes outbreaks, and practicing safer sex in between?

Opening up about herpes can be intimidating, and certainly there are individuals who choose *not* to tell a sex partner about herpes or who find it impossible to tell until after they've had sex. There are countless combinations of people and circumstances, and no book such as this can presume to anticipate them all. In couples who pursue an ongoing relationship, however, it's clearly helpful if herpes isn't a secret locked away from your lover.

For one thing, the secrecy itself is likely to cause more anxiety than telling the truth. The closer you become, the more you'll want to be honest—yet the task at hand is likely to get harder over time. If and when you do finally disclose the truth, suddenly there are two issues on the table. One is herpes. But potentially more explosive is the issue of trust.

Withholding the truth has other disadvantages as well. It puts the entire burden of preventing the spread of herpes on one person. It may also lead to the adoption of unhealthy or irrational strategies to avert outbreaks or avoid sex, such as making up stories to explain away times when you cannot be intimate. These strategies themselves can be quite stressful and actually make having herpes more of a burden than it would otherwise be.

There also are ethical and legal implications. Everyone has the right to make an informed choice about his or her sexual partner, and the courts have ruled in some cases that failure to disclose a sexually transmitted infection like herpes may be grounds for a lawsuit. (These suits aren't common, but some individuals do choose to bring legal action.)

It's clear that keeping herpes secret from your lover can fuel emotional stress, but there are health-related issues at stake as well. Just as your partner may be at risk for herpes, he or she may place you at risk for a number of other STDs. *You* have something to gain from knowing your potential partner's sexual history, too. So it makes sense to talk about herpes in the context of overall sexual health. This approach equalizes people from the beginning. Remember also that about one-fifth of the adult population has herpes, though most don't know it. So a potential partner may have the same virus. (Herpes diagnostic tests for partners are discussed in chapters 12 and 16.)

In reality, questions about risks to your health are relevant to both partners: Have you had another lover in the past? Have you used condoms? Have you ever had a sexually transmitted disease? Do you realize that you can have HIV or other STDs and not know it? These may be difficult issues to raise, but frank discussion about these things is becoming the norm in more relationships all the time.

Honesty and open communication not only pave the way for making smart choices about prevention, they also carry emotional benefits, not the least of which are mutual trust and respect. Sometimes the person who is newly diagnosed feels reluctant to tell anyone about herpes. But psychologists have found that telling a sexual partner is very important in making the adjustment to herpes and learning to cope with it. Herpes or no herpes, communication and sharing are two of the cornerstones for any successful relationship. What's more, behavioral research has shown that the most effective emotional support for people with herpes comes from their lovers or close friends.

STARTING WITH YOURSELF

Once you've decided to tell a partner about herpes, it may prove helpful to think through the process and anticipate some of the potential issues.

First, it's important to consider whether you've come to terms with herpes yourself and accepted that it's not such an earth-shaking problem. There's little to gain from opening up to others about herpes if you're likely to characterize it in the most negative way or if you are still punishing yourself over it in some way.

Self-image is a relevant concern here. If herpes has radically altered the way you see yourself, it may be the best first step is to consider why herpes is affecting you and then try to address the root of the problem. Perhaps a trusted friend or counselor could help you think through these issues.

Whether or not you find it necessary to assess your self-esteem in this way, it's a good idea to know the key facts about herpes and feel comfortable discussing them. Be prepared for a range of questions—some of them thought-provoking and some of them quite simple. You probably know a great deal by now, but you have to assume that your audience is starting from scratch.

PREPARING TO TELL: WHEN AND HOW

Each person will have a style and presentation that's unique, and no one should feel constrained to use a schedule or a script that just doesn't fit the situation. However you proceed, though, your attitude and your mood will have a great deal of influence on how the news is received. People tend to behave the way you expect them to behave, and a gloomy presentation may well increase the chance of a gloomy response. So the key is: be positive and be confident. Expect that your partner will be accepting and supportive. You are doing the right thing for both of you.

What's the best time? People who have shared their experiences through herpes support groups or the newsletters of the National Herpes Resource Center tend to agree that it's usually best to allow a relationship to develop a bit before bringing up the subject. A conversation about sexual health is going to be easier if you have begun to feel comfortable with someone and safe about being honest.

If you do become interested in someone and begin to feel comfortable in the relationship, you can prepare yourself and look for logical opportunities to broach the subject. A television or newspaper report on sexual health—infertility or AIDS, for instance—might naturally start a conversation about safer sex.

A passionate embrace, however, is definitely not the perfect opportunity it might seem to be. In the heat of a sexually charged moment, discussion of herpes or other STDs can be particularly awkward and frustrating. Your partner may be angry with you for spoiling the mood, and this may color the entire conversation. Likewise, it's probably best not to broach the subject en route to a romantic getaway.

Many people choose to plan carefully a time and place for the conversation. And the consensus is that talking to a partner about sexual history works best when both individuals feel good, are relaxed, and can devote their full attention to the conversation. The place should be private. It could be your own home or a quiet outdoor setting—anywhere that's relatively free of interruptions.

WHAT TO SAY

If you're worried about how to handle the situation, you may want to write down what amounts to a script and practice it. Knowing what to say and actually speaking the words in advance can make things easier when the time comes.

Clearly, people take countless approaches, but a number of common elements are often cited:

> • Begin the conversation by pointing to the strengths of the relationship. For example: "I really feel I can trust you, and I'd like to tell you something very personal. Last year I found out I had contracted genital herpes." Or: "I really enjoy being with you, and I'm starting to feel very safe with you. It seems possible we will want to be more intimate in the future, so I think it's time we talk about safer sex."

> • In describing herpes, keep things in perspective. Stress that it's a common viral infection and that there's medication available to treat it. Many people like to make the comparison with cold sores, since these are acknowledged as a very minor concern. For example: "Have you ever

had a cold sore or a fever blister? The reason I ask is that cold sores are caused by a type of virus—herpes simplex virus. I have this virus, only for me instead of causing a sore on the lips, it can cause one below the waist."

• Mention that most people have either HSV-1 or HSV-2, and about one in five adults has genital herpes. It's usually so mild, however, that many people don't know they have it. Even people who have received a "clean bill of health" from a doctor or STD clinic may have undiagnosed genital herpes, since most standard blood tests are unreliable for detecting HSV-2.

• In the interest of full disclosure, explain that herpes can be spread during sexual contact when sores or other symptoms are present. There may also be a risk of transmission at other times, but a person can take precautions to lower this risk.

Whatever the script, it's crucial to avoid being over-dramatic. Remember: your delivery affects your message. Try to be calm and confident, straightforward and sincere. Frame the conversation the way you've decided to, and avoid language that's inherently negative. Lastly, don't lose sight of the fact that you want a dialogue, so it's best not to go on at great length. You want to discuss the issue, not lecture or confess.

Some may simply need time to process what you've said. Other times the first response is an attempt to sort out the information, and some people will want to read something on herpes, such as a brochure or book. Remember: you may have known very little about herpes before you were diagnosed. In any case, you have everything to gain from helping to provide information. You can also give a partner the telephone number of the National Herpes Hotline.

Having a partner take matters under advisement or go elsewhere for information isn't easy, but it's reasonable to expect that someone who is new to the idea of herpes may need time to absorb the facts and check their own feelings. And the outcome can be very satisfying, as in the case of Lauren. "I contracted herpes five years ago from a partner who failed to tell me that he had it," she writes. "I have slowly come to terms with my anger towards him and myself. Since that time, I have been sexually active with two different men. Each time, I chose to talk about herpes *before* getting sexually involved. In each case, my boyfriend decided that herpes should not get in the way of having a sexual relationship. Both needed time or needed to read something before making a decision, and one consulted his doctor. My point is simply that it may take some patience, but you can have this conversation and have it turn out well."

Also, remain open to the possibility that the person you're talking to may have herpes themselves. In describing the disease, you may have cited the fact that herpes goes unrecognized most of the time. The person you're telling may be one of those who has this type of unrecognized infection. In approaching the subject, make sure the person understands you are not implying he or she has herpes already or accusing them of withholding information from you. On the other hand, if the relationship progresses, getting a type-specific blood test for herpes can establish whether you and your potential partner already have the same type of HSV. If so, you may decide that there's less need to take precautions between outbreaks. We'll discuss these tests and their use further in Chapter 12 and Chapter 16.

Clearly, if there are countless approaches, there are an equal number of subtleties in the responses you might get. Some people may overreact, some won't bat an eye. Given the number of people who have herpes, many will have had this discussion before. Whatever the reaction, try to be flexible yourself. Remember that it took you time to adjust as well, and that the first response is not always the one that counts.

At the same time, some experts say, don't be overly concerned about protecting the feelings of your partner. Yes, you want him or her to have the time needed to process this information. But after all, you have needs yourself. And you probably don't need a relationship in which you have to do all the emotional work. Has your partner given you a feeling of emotional support? It's important to assess the other person's behavior when presented with the challenge of a safer sex discussion. People who are judgmental, those who have a very narrow life experience, or those who are obsessive about germs may not be the best candidates for your love.

The majority of people will react well. After all, you trust them enough to share a confidence with them that you probably wouldn't share with just anybody. Most people respect that. And in talking about safer sex, you've shown maturity in facing up to a health issue of mutual importance for any two people. So, when you talk to someone about herpes and safer sex, pat yourself on the back. You have confronted a difficult issue in your life with courage and consideration.

12

HERPES AND
YOUR SEX LIFE

◯

"I've been in a stable relationship for over a year," says Denise. "At first I didn't know how to tell him I had herpes, but through an unplanned conversation about past lovers and STDs he learned about it. He has since been very understanding, sympathetic, and supportive. Our relationship has grown into one of deeper commitment and trust. We work to keep communication open, and I'm learning to share my concerns about herpes with him, including my fear that he will eventually get it.

"To be honest, I still dread bringing up herpes when I'm having prodrome or suspect lesions, but it's better to talk to him about it than to have the fears and just avoid sexual intimacy."

People do worry about the effect herpes is going to have on their sex life. It's one of the concerns that can make herpes seem so devastating initially, and it's central to the anxiety over telling a partner. Starting or maintaining an intimate relationship isn't the easiest thing in the world, anyway. And putting herpes into the mix seems at first to add an unwanted layer of complexity.

In assessing its likely impact on one's sex life, it's useful to remember that herpes affects everyone differently at an emotional level. For some, it's a minor matter. For others, it can cause a number of concerns, including problems of self-esteem or feelings of isolation. Sexually, it can affect one's sense of spontaneity or freedom. Some may feel more hesitant to approach new partners or may experience a decrease in sexual pleasure around the time of diagnosis—feelings that often center on the fear of spreading herpes to a partner. These concerns may be heightened if the person is experiencing frequent outbreaks.

As with other aspects of genital herpes, however, such concerns tend to be especially pressing in the first few months after being diagnosed. Later, they tend to fade. In fact, one study found that there were no long-term changes in the sex lives of persons diagnosed with herpes, compared with the period before diagnosis. In the first six months, study participants recalled concerns such as decreased frequency of sexual activity. But over time those surveyed enjoyed sex, functioned well, and were just as sexually active as they had been before being diagnosed.

Talking about the lessening impact of herpes over the long term is not to trivialize it or deny that it may bring some changes to your sex life. The most important of these is probably the issue of risk reduction—of protecting sexual partners.

The desire to protect a sexual partner and prevent the spread of herpes is often very strong. In a number of different studies, a very high percentage of people with herpes listed fear of infecting a partner as one of their primary concerns. In this chapter we'll take a detailed look at the factors that increase or lower the risk of transmitting herpes and at the steps you can take to reduce this risk in your relationships. We'll also review considerations that may influence these choices, such as the possibility that your sexual partner wants to be tested for herpes. Testing, after all, can color this entire discussion. If you and a partner have the same type of HSV, the risk of transmission becomes moot and the precautions listed here may be irrelevant in this particular relationship.

THE BASICS

First we'll focus on herpes by itself. Forget about whether you're gay or straight, coupled or single; forget about the other STDs. In the absence of all other factors, what you can do to prevent the spread of herpes boils down to two steps: (1) avoid direct skin-to-skin contact with herpes lesions during obvious flare-ups; and (2) use condoms or take other precautions between outbreaks as a guard against the asymptomatic shedding discussed in earlier chapters.

Both of these issues center on times when HSV has reactivated and caused the process of viral shedding. The period during which you're actually contagious may in fact be a relatively small percentage of the time. Because being contagious is unpredictable, however, the precautions needed to protect a partner deserve a detailed discussion.

During Outbreaks

The risk of spreading herpes is highest whenever symptoms, ranging from subtle to painful, are present. The tingling or itch of prodrome, for example, is a signal that virus has probably found its way to the skin and that there is risk of spreading HSV to a sexual partner. An itchy red patch of skin near the genitals also should be considered a likely site of viral shedding, as should a classic herpes blister. Herpes can be spread when any such signs and symptoms are present.

Sometimes a person may experience the symptoms of prodrome and then have no visible signs of infection at all. This is sometimes called a "false prodrome," but it can just as easily be regarded as a minor outbreak. You should still consider that the risk of transmission is high when the itching or tingling sensations occur, because the virus may be present on your skin at this time.

When signs and symptoms are present, any direct genital-to-genital contact or sexual act that involves penetration, such as vaginal or anal sex, create a high risk of transmission. Also included as risky would be oral-to-genital contact (mouth on vaginal area or mouth on penis), because of the direct contact between mucous membranes.

When can you consider an outbreak over? The basic rule is to avoid direct contact with the affected area from the first hint of prodrome until any skin lesions are fully healed and the skin surface looks normal again. In some cases, this is a matter of days. With recurrences, the process takes 4 to 6 days on average; with a first episode, it may be quite a bit longer. Studies have shown that asymptomatic shedding is most probable in the days immediately before or after an outbreak, so after herpes lesions heal—even after a scab falls off—it's safest to leave the tender new skin alone for a few days.

What about simply using condoms during outbreaks? Unfortunately, condoms do not offer complete protection during these periods. There are a variety of possible reasons for this. Incorrect or inconsistent use is certainly a major factor. A complete discussion of condom dos and don'ts is included in the next chapter. In addition, in terms of simple geography, some herpes lesions will be covered or protected by a condom, but some will not. A herpes lesion on the upper thigh, for example, will not be covered. Alternately if a woman were having a lesion in the folds of the vulva or in the perianal area, it's unclear whether the use of a condom by a male partner would provide complete coverage and protection.

All of this would be much simpler, too, if an outbreak were always a matter of a lesion you could clearly see. In reality, however, during recurrences HSV may travel to several skin sites at once. There may be an obvious lesion in one place—say, on the penis—and asymptomatic shedding in another.

In summary, condoms might help reduce the risk of transmission during outbreaks, depending on the circumstances. But they are not a guarantee of protection.

While the risk of spreading herpes is high when lesions are present, some couples find creative ways to give one another pleasure without taking large risks. First, as long as there are no lesions on the mouth, kissing poses no risk. Sensual massage, mutual masturbation, fantasy—all these are sexual practices that some people recount using as forms of risk reduction, and many say they are quite pleasurable.

Many people wonder about risks involved in use of the hands for sexual pleasuring. No form of skin-to-skin contact with a herpes lesion is absolutely risk-free. For example, HSV could be transferred from a site of viral shedding to an uninfected partner during lovemaking by way of the hand. In a ranking of risks, use of the hands is probably safer than genital-to-genital contact or oral sex, because the thick skin of the hands is less vulnerable to

HSV. When lesions are present, however, concern about transmission via the hands is warranted.

Refraining from intercourse isn't easy sometimes, and in one recent study, about one-fifth of couples in monogamous relationships reported that they sometimes chose to have intercourse when lesions were present. It's clear, however, that a greater number of exposures to herpes lesions increases the risk of transmission. Therefore, couples who refrain from sexual intercourse during outbreaks are taking an important step to avoid spreading herpes from one to the other.

Between Outbreaks

Even if you have outbreaks more often than the average person, the vast majority of your life will be symptom-free. The problem is the issue of asymptomatic viral shedding.

As we noted earlier, asymptomatic shedding is at its peak in the six months immediately after a first episode. During this time, asymptomatic shedding will occur on an average of 6% of days. (In one large study, shedding rates ranged from 0% to 25%.) Afterwards, asymptomatic shedding rates range from 0% to 10%. The average works out to be about 4% of days, something on the order of two weeks out of the year. The problem is, you don't know which days these will be.

What can you do about it? For straight or gay couples practicing vaginal or anal intercourse, experts say that the most thorough approach is to use condoms between outbreaks. You recall that condoms were *not* recommended as protection *during* outbreaks, but they're considered a better bet for asymptomatic shedding. Why? Research to date suggests that the biggest risk of asymptomatic transmission occurs when there is contact between surfaces such as the penis or the soft mucosal tissue of the vagina, cervix, or anus. And these, of course, are among the areas which *tend to be* covered or protected by condoms.

The best overall data we have about condoms comes from a recent vaccine study, which followed several hundred couples over a period of time and documented each instance where herpes was spread from one partner to the other. In this study, condom use was quite low in spite of the fact that all participants were counseled to use them consistently. But results showed that those who used condoms for the largest percentage of sexual acts did have a significantly reduced risk of transmission.

Though research is still pending, another potential approach to lowering the risk of transmission during times of asymptomatic shedding is to use suppressive therapy. Daily use of antivirals has been shown to reduce asymptomatic shedding by 80% to 94%, and further studies to see if antivirals reduce the risk of transmission are under way.

RISK REDUCTION FOR GAYS AND LESBIANS

The sparse data that have been gathered about the transmission of herpes stem primarily from research on heterosexual couples, but gays and lesbians often raise questions about the particular risks they may face. In addition, many people—both straight and gay—are eager to learn whether anything is known about the relative risks of various sexual acts.

Unfortunately, medical science has little to say about the probability of transmission through oral sex versus anal versus other types of sexual pleasuring. But there are some insights about herpes that may be particularly pertinent for gays and for lesbians.

Given the enormous impact of AIDS, people in the gay community are better informed about HIV prevention than most other segments of the U.S. population. The importance of herpes and other STDs as risk factors for acquiring HIV, however, has not always been well publicized. Specifically, research has shown that genital herpes—and, in fact, a number of other STDs—create tiny breaks in the skin and in mucosal tissue that give HIV a portal of entry. In addition, herpes lesions attract larger than average numbers of T-cells—precisely the kind of lymphocyte that HIV likes to attack. Given these two factors, the person who is experiencing a herpes outbreak or an episode of asymptomatic shedding has an especially high risk of getting infected with HIV if he or she is exposed to HIV. The "if" here is important, because it is not true that herpes puts one on some inevitable path to HIV. But the added risk of HIV is worth considering. For similar reasons, those who are HIV-positive and also have genital herpes are likely more efficient transmitters of HIV as well.

All of the above argues for the same kinds of precautions outlined previously, such as abstaining from sex during outbreaks and condom use at other times. Condoms have been studied more thoroughly for their efficacy in vaginal sex, but for over a decade the Centers for Disease Control and Prevention has been recommending their use for anal and oral sex as well. For anal sex, water-based lubricants will likely offer an extra measure of protection, decreasing the likelihood of condom breakage and of trauma to the rectum that can result from anal intercourse.

In contrast to the situation with gay men, lesbians have been regarded as unlikely to acquire STDs such as herpes and HIV. But while the rates of some STDs are indeed lower in lesbians, a recent study at the University of Washington showed that some 13% of lesbian women tested positive for HSV-2. How do they acquire it? First, researchers point out that as many as 90% of women who identify themselves as lesbian have had sex with men at some point in their lives. Second, given the importance of oral sex in lesbian couples, it's likely that HSV is sometimes spread through oral-genital contact, and likely as well that there is a fairly high percentage of HSV-1 in lesbian women that represents latent genital infection. Third, women who have sex with women may be able to transmit STDs such as genital HPV—and possibly herpes—through sex toys and through use of the hands for pleasuring.

In terms of prevention, researchers stress that women who have sex with women should be aware that oral sex does pose a risk of transmission. In this regard, as a barrier during oral sex, some women use household plastic wrap as protective barrier and some use nonpowdered latex gloves, which can be cut to a suitable flat shape for covering the vulva. As far as for sex toys, it's important to understand that viruses or bacteria deposited on the toy by one person can infect the other during penetration or rubbing. The best advice, therefore, is to clean them with soap and water before sharing.

SELF-IMAGE AND SEXUAL GROWTH

A great deal has been written on the practicalities of "safer sex." A lot of it, unfortunately, doesn't get to the heart of the matter for many people who have recently been diagnosed and are feeling very threatened by the potential changes in their sexual habits.

In the ASHA survey, for example, many respondents noted ways in which herpes affected their sense of sexual spontaneity or freedom. Some felt more hesitant to approach new partners, while a few withdrew from sexual activity for months or even years. Two out of three said they experienced a decrease in sexual pleasure around the time of diagnosis. And almost as many reported that herpes lessened sexual drive during outbreaks. Similar results were found in a number of studies over the past 15 years.

As with other aspects of genital herpes, however, for many individuals the impact on sexuality lessens markedly over time. One researcher noted that after a period of six months, persons diagnosed with herpes were enjoying sex just as much as they did before and functioned just as they had before. In the short term, however, one may experience a sense of loss in having to feel more constrained in one's sex life. Frequently, a period of adjustment—even a period of mourning—may be needed.

At the same time, it can be very damaging to conclude that you're no longer a sexual person or no longer allowed to express sexual desire. STDs such as herpes sometimes have the seeming power to overwhelm us and become what psychologists call "master status traits." Thus, our sexual self-image can undergo a change because of a medical condition.

If you're feeling this way, it may be important to keep sight of the fact that millions of people with herpes do have satisfying sexual relationships. When questioned about the long-term impact of herpes, counselors and sex therapists point out that a condition like genital herpes can actually have a very positive effect on relationships. Talking through an issue like herpes can create a deeper level of trust and intimacy, and some couples say that herpes influences them to explore and grow sexually.

Herpes can press couples to communicate about what is sexually pleasing. And that's no small accomplishment, because people in all sorts of relationships often have trouble talking about sex. Needs and desires remain unspoken out of embarrassment. But being forced to speak about them can have unforeseen benefits and result in more mature and more creative sex.

An easy way to begin communicating about sex is to tell your partner you want to talk about it. Talking about "talking about" sex can lead a couple to share their fears and feelings. They may then be comfortable enough to begin an ongoing process of sexual communication.

Says one therapist: "I've had clients who have had to deal with severe herpes outbreaks over time. But it's not really an issue. A satisfying sexuality really has more to do with being comfortable with sexuality in general, being able to talk about it with your partner, and being willing to try new things with your partner. Healthy sexuality has more to do with the couple's *attitude* about sex than it has to do with an issue such as herpes."

If all the talk about condoms puts you off, or if you've been diagnosed recently and are just not ready to become sexually active, remember two things: First, it may take a while before you feel yourself again, but you're still a whole and healthy individual who can have satisfying sexual relationships. Second, you may discover new aspects of your sexuality because of herpes.

THINKING THROUGH THE ISSUES:
TESTING, RISK, AND CHOICES

Faced with all this information, many people understandably have a hard time knowing what to do about herpes and sex. Unfortunately, this book can't provide any easy answers or foolproof formulas. Every person has a unique situation and unique set of values, and decisions about sex hinge on both.

In addition, it's worth mentioning again that, while a person with herpes may be highly concerned about their partner, they should not be oblivious to the need to protect themselves from other, potentially more serious sexually transmitted infections. As we've said, there are 15 million new sexually transmitted infections each year, and some experts say that 50% of adults—whatever their race, sex, or social class—will have an STD at some point. Many of these infections can remain hidden, so that those who carry them don't know about it. The point is that while protecting a partner is often the focal point for safer sex practices, the person with herpes should not overlook their own risk. In many circumstances, personal risk will or should influence one's decision, for example, on condom use.

In terms of protecting a partner against herpes, the first issue is: does your partner possibly have herpes already? As we mentioned earlier, this may not be an easy matter to bring up, and you would want to avoid any implication that your partner is withholding something from you. However, if your partner has learned the basics about herpes, understands how widespread it is, and understands that up to 90% of those who have antibodies don't recognize symptoms, then it may make sense to talk about testing. If the two of you agree that it's important to find out, you can get one of the new "type-specific" blood tests for HSV. Then, if your partner already has the same type of herpes you do, you may decide that there's less need to take precautions between outbreaks. Finding an accurate test and learning more about how to interpret the test are two topics covered in detail in Chapter 16.

If testing is not an option, or if you discover that your partner does not have herpes, there are several aspects of risk reduction to consider. First, it's clear that the highest risk of transmission occurs when symptoms are present. So most couples will choose either to refrain from sex during outbreaks or to engage in sexual activities that are relatively safe.

When it comes to the periods between outbreaks, however, it's often harder to know what to do. Do you use condoms all the time or practice some other form of safer sex? What we've tried to stress is that people who have several sexual partners or a casual relationship have many reasons to practice safer sex in any case. Regular condom use, for example, often makes sense in these situations. For people in a monogamous relationship, the choice is more complicated. In making this decision, people sometimes want to know the precise odds that a partner will become infected.

Science can only go so far in determining "how safe" or "how risky" any sexual behavior might be, but there are a few factors that appear to affect "the odds." Researchers, for example, have studied the rate of transmission in heterosexual couples in which one partner has herpes and one does not. The average rate appears to be about 10% per year, and the most recent data suggests that this rate can be significantly lowered if couples use condoms between outbreaks. The more that condoms are used, it appears, the lower the risk of transmission.

You may find in the scientific literature a number of papers that show differences between men and women in the risk of acquiring genital HSV. Some studies suggest that women are up to six times as likely as men to become infected with herpes if exposed to the virus. A similar increase in risk to women is noted with several other STDs as well. At least in part, this is probably due to the physical differences between the sexes—mainly the presence of more mucosal tissue in women. In any case, the data on condoms and the higher risk faced by women both point to the fact that an uninfected woman might benefit greatly from regular condom use.

Recent research has also turned up new insights into other risk factors as well. It appears that risk of transmission is highest when the person with herpes has both HSV-1 and HSV-2. Risk is also increased early in the course of a sexual relationship. The most obvious explanation for this is the fact that couples tend to have sex more often early in the relationship, and the number of exposures correlates with increased risk. Some scientists also theorize that transmission rates are higher early on because people vary in how easily they get the infection. In this hypothesis, the first year may sort out the "susceptibles" from those who are not.

How big a factor is transmission during episodes of asymptomatic shedding? Clinical studies find couples in which one partner has herpes and one does not—even after several years together. They also find couples in which a person with herpes has passed the infection to a partner *despite* having refrained from sex during outbreaks. For this reason they recommend that couples understand and talk about the issue of asymptomatic shedding and the advisibility of using condoms between outbreaks.

Another matter worth mentioning is drug therapy. If your herpes flare-ups are frequent and are posing problems in an important relationship, you might consider suppressive therapy with an antiviral drug. As noted here and in Chapter 9, a daily dose of an antiviral drug can completely halt outbreaks in many people. The use of suppressive medication cannot guarantee you'll be completely free of asymptomatic shedding and should not be considered a sole form of prevention, but it can affect the pattern of recurrent outbreaks and asymptomatic shedding as well. It's something you may want to discuss with your healthcare provider.

In some relationships, risk reduction won't be a major issue. You may have a partner who knows there is a chance of becoming infected but simply is not worried about it. Alternately you may find your partner has the same type of HSV already, and you may decide that there is less need to take precautions between outbreaks.

In cases where couples both have some form of HSV, various questions can arise. If two partners both have genital HSV-2, for example, is there any need for precautions? For the most part, no. In this scenario, however, experts would still recommend avoiding sex when symptoms are present, because it's possible—though unlikely—to be reinfected with a different strain of HSV-2.

Some couples also wonder what to do when one person has a history of type 1 herpes (say cold sores) and the other a history of genital herpes. Will each of them become infected with both types? And will they have more frequent recurrences as a result?

The research on this question has produced contradictory

findings. Some studies suggest that the person with pre-existing HSV-1 infection has a lower risk of acquiring HSV-2. Others, however, find little or no protective effect. On the other hand, it seems clear that the person with pre-existing HSV-2 does have some protection against HSV-1. So the body's natural defenses are at least partially relevant. In addition, one might weigh the "sites of preference" argument—that is, even if one becomes infected with genital HSV-1, recurrences are less frequent than they are with genital HSV-2. Recurrences of oral HSV-2 are even rarer.

Some couples in long-term relationships find that they are less concerned about the possibility of transmission as time goes on. Some couples who have transmitted herpes after many years even report a feeling of relief, as the worry about transmitting herpes proved more troublesome than genital herpes itself. Again, how couples respond to herpes in a long-term relationship depends upon many individual factors.

In the end, genital herpes doesn't have to stand in the way of having a healthy and satisfying sex life. Taking precautions to protect your partner—and to protect yourself from other STDs—is something that more and more people are learning to negotiate. There are as many different approaches as there are different people. Just keep in mind that there is more to safer sex than latex or spermicides. Trust and communication lie at the center of any healthy relationship.

13

CONDOMS, SPERMICIDES, MICROBICIDES, AND MORE

The standard male condom found in almost any drug store is an effective form of STD prevention. Many studies, including those among couples in which one partner is HIV-infected and the other is not, have proved that condoms offer a high degree of protection against HIV, the most dangerous STD. Solid research has also demonstrated condoms' effectiveness against gonorrhea, the most easily transmitted STD. A government report released by the National Institutes of Health in 2001 noted a lack of rigorous studies on the role of condoms against several other common sexually transmitted infections, including chlamydia and trichomoniasis. However, the report cited growing evidence for condoms in preventing genital warts and cervical infection related to genital human papillomavius (HPV), an STD similar in some ways to herpes. In addition, a published study subsequent to the NIH report showed condoms offer significant protection against genital herpes as well.

Used correctly, condoms also can prevent pregnancy. Condoms have a 14% failure rate in "typical use," which reflects the percentage of couples which become pregnant while using condoms over the course of a full year. While there is potential for user error with this method, condoms actually have lower failure rates in typical use than diaphragms, cervical caps, and several other contraceptive methods.

Condoms are widely available and, for the most part, easy to use, but there are a few important points worth reviewing.

USING CONDOMS

When it comes to STD protection, any condom is better than none, but condoms made of latex or plastic (polyurethane) are better than those made of animal membrane. Latex condoms are superior to plastic condoms, but for people allergic to latex, plastic condoms are a reasonable alternative. "Lambskin" or animal-membrane condoms have pores large enough to admit some viruses—at least in laboratory experiments—and are not recommended for maximal STD protection. Even the smallest viruses cannot permeate latex or plastic. Condoms sold for contraception and disease protection in this country are classified as medical devices. They are regulated by the U.S. Food and Drug Administration and carefully tested and inspected during the manufacturing process. Every latex condom sold in the U.S. is tested electronically for holes before packaging. Condom failure usually results from inconsistent or incorrect use rather than condom breakage.

Latex is recommended by public health authorities as the preferred type of condom for STD protection. Two randomized, controlled studies comparing latex condoms and plastic condoms have shown that latex condoms are less likely than plastic condoms to break or slip off during use. In the larger of these two studies the failure rate, including breaking or slipping during intercourse or withdrawal, was 8.5% with the plastic condom versus 1.6% with the latex condom. Men were generally more satisfied with the latex condom, and more men dropped out of the study because of problems with the plastic condom.

If you are starting to use condoms for the first time, it's important to review the package insert or other written instructions about how to use them correctly. The basics are as follows:

- Condoms should be stored in a cool, dry place out of direct sunlight—no wallets or glove compartments.

- Put the condom on before any genital contact occurs. If the condom has a reservoir tip, squeeze the tip closed and unroll the condom onto the erect penis. Air bubbles may lead to breakage.

- If the condom does not have a reservoir tip, hold the end of the condom between the thumb and the forefinger and unroll the condom onto the erect penis. This should leave extra room at the tip of the condom (to hold semen after ejaculation).

- Unroll the condom to cover the entire erect penis. The unrolled ring should be on the outside. If the condom is on inside out, do not flip it over. Use another one.

- *If the condom is latex,* only water-based lubricants should be used (K-Y® Brand Jelly, Replens®, or Astroglide®, for example). Oil-based lubricants can damage latex, so do not use Vaseline® petroleum jelly, baby oil, vegetable oil, or most hand and skin lotions.

• *If the condom is plastic,* the oil-based lubricants mentioned above will not degrade the material.

• Following ejaculation, while the penis is still erect, hold the base of the condom and withdraw, taking care not to let the condom slip off. A condom should never be used twice.

Condoms can be used for various sexual activities. They are tested under conditions that simulate vaginal intercourse, but some experts consider them effective for oral sex and anal sex as well. Condoms can be used with or without lubricant. Many brands are coated with lubricant at the factory, though unlubricated brands are also available. Because many people object to the smell and taste of latex, some manufacturers also market flavored condoms specifically for use in oral sex.

In fact, because of the emphasis on safer sex beginning in the late 1980s, condom manufacturers actually have been quite busy developing new models. In addition to the plastic condom recently developed for men, there are a number of condoms designed to be used by women. One type of female condom (branded as Reality® or The Female Condom™) resembles a pouch with a flexible loop on either end. The smaller of the two loops is inserted in the vagina, covering the cervix, and the larger loop lies outside, covering the vulva. It was hoped this model might actually offer greater protection against STDs than the standard male condom because it covers more area, but so far we have no conclusive evidence that it is more protective. In any case, it gives women an option they can initiate. Some women whose partners cannot or will not use latex condoms are able to use the female condom.

As we noted, male condoms can be used for oral sex, but obviously this is practical only for oral sex performed on a man. For oral sex performed on a woman, you may have read about the use of a latex barrier such as a *dental dam* to block direct contact between the mouth and the vulva. Unfortunately, dental dams (rectangular latex sheets used in oral surgery) are fairly small and are thicker than condoms, making them impractical at best. In addition, they're seldom available at retail stores. An alternative that has advantages over latex is plastic household food wrap. This can be cut in a larger sheet and used to cover more area. Some couples use this sort of barrier for cunnilingus.

SPERMICIDES & MICROBICIDES

People concerned about safer sex often ask questions about spermicide as well. The active ingredient in foams, jellies, and suppositories used by some women to prevent pregnancy also kills or disables certain viruses and bacteria. It turns out that HSV is one of the viruses that can be disabled by spermicide, at least in the laboratory.

For a number of practical reasons, however, experts caution against relying too much on spermicide as protection against any STD, particularly genital herpes. For one thing, spermicide is effective only when a full dose is used. That means using the amount required by the package instructions for contraceptive purposes.

Secondly, spermicide effectiveness depends on direct contact with the virus. If the inside of the vagina is coated with spermicide, some protection is offered to the cervix and interior of the vagina as well as to the shaft and head of the penis. But, as we've seen with condoms, herpes lesions and herpes shedding may occur in places where there simply isn't any barrier of spermicide.

Lastly, there is evidence that spermicides help to stop infections like chlamydia and gonorrhea. But there is also some evidence that spermicides, if used frequently, may irritate the vagina, causing tiny breaks in the tissue that may invite other infections. As a result, the active compound in most spermicidal products, nonoxynol-9, is no longer recommended as protection against HIV infection.

Condoms coated with a spermicide might make claims for better effectiveness in disease prevention, but this, too, is a matter of speculation. There's probably too little spermicide present to offer much protection.

New research on compounds called microbicides that are specifically designed to kill sexually transmitted germs and viruses may produce a superior alternative to the spermicides developed as contraceptives. For now, however, a good rule of thumb for spermicides and STDs generally is this: Spermicides may offer some extra protection against infection when used *along with* condoms, but they should not be used in place of condoms.

CONDOMS IN CONTEXT

Many couples who understand the risk of unrecognized herpes reactivation ask the question: Should everyone use condoms between outbreaks? This is a decision that will be made ideally as a couple, depending on the individuals and their circumstances. The following scenarios illustrate two possibilities:

LOOKING FOR LOVE

Diane is in her mid-20s. She got herpes from someone she dated when she was just out of college. The relationship ended some time ago. She's dated a couple of people since then but hasn't had sex with any of them. Now she's interested in Roger, and she's told him about having herpes. He still wants to get involved, but he doesn't know quite what to do about protection.

Diane suggests they shouldn't have sex when she's having an outbreak, which is three or four times a year. Also, she has lived with her herpes long enough to know when an outbreak is coming, so she's never caught by surprise. Still, she wonders about unrecognized herpes reactivation.

She also wonders about Roger's past history. He's had several partners before her, and he's never been tested for any sexually transmitted infection.

After considering the risks for both of them, they decide they will become sexually intimate, but they choose to use condoms every time they're together and to refrain from sex when Diane has symptoms.

The characters here could be younger or older, straight, gay, or bisexual. With HIV around, however, there is good reason to know your partner's sexual history, and good reason to use condoms.

Of course, there also are situations in which people don't make choices as a couple and may not have the benefit of knowing a partner's past history. In the proverbial "one-night stand," a person is well-advised to use condoms or practice some form of safer sex. The choice to "just take the risk" and ignore the need for protection is often one that people come to regret.

THE STEADY RELATIONSHIP

Back to Diane and Roger. They're still together a year later and have decided to move in together. They both want the relationship to last, and they figure it probably will. Roger has begun to question why they're using condoms. He's seen that Diane has very little problem with herpes, and he wonders whether it's worth the trouble of taking precautions between outbreaks. So they talk about it. Diane says she's not worried about getting an STD from Roger, and they trust each other. Still, they feel it would be best if they both get checked out for some of the other sexually transmitted diseases that can hang around for years but cause no symptoms.

In the end, they both get a "clean bill of health," and they decide together that they'll stop using condoms in between outbreaks, but put off sex when symptoms are present. They know there is some risk with herpes, but they're in love, and they're willing to take it.

There are many possible variations here, of course. Roger may have been determined to avoid getting herpes, or Diane may have been determined to avoid transmitting it, and therefore, they may have preferred to stick with condoms. Or either partner may have had a sexual relationship with someone else in the meantime, raising the possibility of a new STD. Or Diane and Roger might have decided to try to conceive a child, which would place condom use in a wholly different light.

Whatever the variation, the point is that couples in which one member has herpes must weigh the risks of spreading herpes, along with all the other issues they face. Some people truly find genital herpes so trivial a matter that they're willing to forego condoms altogether, particularly in long-term relationships. For others, the use of condoms or other safer sex practices will become an accepted way of life.

MANAGING HERPES

14

HERPES AND PREGNANCY

"After having several outbreaks a year, I got pregnant with my first child," writes Marilu. "And deep down I was really worried. Childbirth was the one thing about herpes that always seemed scary to me. Even so, despite tremendous stress during pregnancy (changing jobs and moving), I had only one outbreak. I delivered vaginally after a long and painful labor. My baby and I were treated with kind and loving care, and after a two-day stay, we went home. My next outbreak occurred a month later."

Even people who have learned to manage genital herpes with ease sometimes have concerns about pregnancy and their ability to give birth to a healthy child. On one hand, these worries are reasonable, because HSV infection in a newborn can be a devastating illness. On the other hand, this kind of herpes infection is quite rare. Out of approximately 4 million live births every year in the United States, the number of babies contracting neonatal herpes is estimated at between one per 3,000 and one per 20,000. In many cases, these babies are born to women who contract herpes late in pregnancy, rather than to women who have long-standing infections. What's more, women who have genital herpes and recognize it can take precautions to lower the already small risk that their infants might become infected.

HOW HSV CAN SPREAD TO NEWBORNS

Transmission of genital HSV to newborns follows the same basic principles that govern transmission between adults and is most likely to occur during labor and delivery. If HSV reactivates in a pregnant woman around the time of labor, it's likely that she will be shedding virus somewhere in the birth canal. Fully developed herpes lesions pose the greatest threat to the infant; therefore, if a woman has signs and symptoms of active herpes infection at labor, precautions are usually taken to protect the baby from infection. Asymptomatic shedding may also pose a risk, especially if it occurs during a first episode.

While the vast majority of transmission from mother to infant takes place at birth, there are two other possibilities. First, researchers believe that in very rare cases a fetus may become infected during pregnancy, especially if the mother has a primary episode during pregnancy. The theory is that a large amount of HSV can be present in the mother's system, and some of it may cross the placenta or find its way into the amniotic fluid. Second, infants can become infected after birth if an adult with active herpes lesions transmits HSV through direct contact. The classic example of this is the relative who has an active cold sore and kisses a baby.

ASSESSING THE RISK

Research on neonatal herpes conducted during the late 1980s has shed a great deal of light on the question of which deliveries carry the highest risk. It turns out that more than half of the babies infected with herpes at delivery are born to mothers who acquired genital herpes in the last few weeks of pregnancy. Some of these women actually had herpes lesions but did not realize it and were not adequately examined before giving birth. Others may have been shedding virus asymptomatically as a result of a first episode. If this seems hard to believe, remember that most people with genital herpes don't know they have it.

In rare cases, babies also can become infected when exposed to asymptomatic viral shedding in the birth canal of mothers who have recurrent genital herpes. In this situation, the risk of transmission to the newborn is quite small—probably less than .01%. When a woman with recurrent herpes has an outbreak at the time of delivery, the risk is much less than with a first episode, but it's still high enough that medical experts recommend delivery by cesarean section (C-section).

Why are the differences between types of herpes infection so dramatic? A herpes infection in a pregnant woman who has never before been infected with HSV-1 or HSV-2 raises the level of risk for four reasons:

1. Neither mother nor infant will have antibodies to HSV.

2. More virus is present in a first episode than in a recurrent outbreak.

3. The cervix is more often involved in a first episode, which means the baby has a greater chance of coming into contact with virus in the birth canal.

4. The virus remains active for a longer period in a first episode.

The relative contribution of each of these factors is not known, but all are thought to play a role in compounding the risk of neonatal infection.

Babies born to women with recurrent genital herpes, on the other hand, have a major advantage over those born to women who first become infected with HSV during pregnancy. Nature offers significant protection to these infants by giving them HSV antibodies while they're still in the womb. These antibodies come directly from the mother and cross the placenta in the blood supply to the fetus. There they can protect the baby from acquiring infection during birth, even if there is virus in the birth canal. Over the first six months of life, as the baby develops its own immune system, these antibodies are gradually lost. Recurrent infection is associated with fewer lesions and is less likely to involve the cervix, and the period of viral shedding is also likely to be shorter than during a first infection.

PREVENTION: WOMEN WITH RECURRENT HERPES

If you are pregnant and have a history of recurrent genital herpes (or recurrent genital symptoms you think may be herpes), the first step is to discuss your medical history with your doctor or midwife. With this information on the table, you and your healthcare provider can make plans for a number of contingencies that may arise if you have an outbreak near the time of labor and delivery. An open discussion of this issue can also help you emotionally by quelling any anxieties you may feel about herpes and an ill-timed recurrence.

The standard of care is to proceed with a normal vaginal

delivery if a woman has no signs or symptoms of an outbreak. If, on the other hand, a woman with recurrent genital herpes has visible lesions or other symptoms of active infection at the time of labor, the baby is delivered by C-section. In this way, the baby is spared the risk of traveling through a birth canal where HSV might be present

If you normally get outbreaks from time to time, you can expect to have some during your pregnancy, particularly in the third trimester. Herpes outbreaks sometimes increase in frequency as pregnancy progresses. There is also a higher than average risk of asymptomatic shedding late in pregnancy. Several years ago, doctors routinely performed viral culture tests on women in their last month of pregnancy to look for viral shedding. They used this information to decide whether to deliver by C-section. However, a number of large studies show that these tests are useless to predict which women are likely to shed virus at the time of labor, and the procedure has been dropped from the guidelines of the American College of Obstetricians and Gynecologists.

What's recommended instead of viral culture is a visual pelvic examination early in labor to look for herpes lesions. Experts point out that in many cases the obstetrician might not be present until late in labor, when the woman's cervix is almost fully dilated. Even then, the standard in many institutions is a quick manual examination. This may prove a case of "too little, too late," because a thorough visual exam with adequate light may be needed to detect herpes lesions. Thus, the need for a visual exam is one of the key issues to bring up with your obstetrician or midwife.

Another point for discussion with your obstetric healthcare provider is C-section delivery. Some women with genital herpes become so concerned about a safe delivery that they urge their doctor or midwife to opt for C-section, and some doctors are inclined to recommend it for similar reasons. Professional concern over malpractice suits also contributes to the high rate of C-section for women with genital herpes. However, leading experts agree that a woman with a history of genital herpes should deliver her baby vaginally unless symptoms (including prodromal symptoms) or herpes sores are present. C-section, they believe, is not needed unless some other complication of pregnancy is also present. The issue is that C-section itself carries a substantial risk and a high cost. C-section is major surgery that entails the health risks of anesthesia, costs several thousand dollars more than a vaginal delivery, and involves a longer and more complicated period of recovery.

In planning for the birth of your baby, it's also important to know the policies of your chosen hospital or birthing center. Some hospitals have very strict procedures for isolating patients whose pregnancy is complicated by infectious disease. Such isolation policies are no longer recommended by herpes experts, but you would be well advised to ask in advance. If the hospital you've chosen has rules that conflict with your plans (plans to "room in," for example), you might want to consider having your baby at a different institution.

Many women wonder about the advisability of taking an antiviral drug during pregnancy to suppress outbreaks in the third trimester. No drug against herpes has been approved for this purpose by the U.S. Food and Drug Administration. Nonetheless, acyclovir is used by some physicians to treat women with genital herpes at the end of pregnancy. Small studies suggest that acyclovir taken daily during the last month of pregnancy will prevent recurrences of genital herpes and, therefore, decrease the need for C-sections, but some experts remain concerned about the safety of fetal exposure to acyclovir.

Besides those cases in which acyclovir has been deliberately prescribed during pregnancy, some women have used it inadvertently before realizing they were expecting. A voluntary registry that tracked both kinds of exposure—more than 1,000 cases— saw no indication that the drug is harmful to mother or child. Still, there is not enough evidence to pronounce the drug categorically safe in pregnancy.

One other issue worth mentioning centers on labor itself. This is the use of fetal scalp monitors. In the largest study to date on herpes and pregnancy, researchers at the University of Washington found that use of this type of monitor appeared to increase the risk of infection. The reason, probably, is that these instruments cause a tiny puncture in the scalp of the fetus, offering a possible opening for virus to enter. The study results weren't conclusive, but experts believe that for women with a history of genital herpes, fetal scalp monitors should be used only when absolutely necessary. An alternative is the external monitor, which tracks the baby's heartbeat through the mother's abdomen. This is a less sensitive instrument and isn't sufficient in all situations, but it carries no risk.

PREVENTION: MEN WITH RECURRENT HERPES

As we've seen, the risk of neonatal herpes is highest when the expectant mother first becomes infected with HSV during late pregnancy. Men can play a critical role in minimizing this risk in some situations. For example, let's look at a common scenario:

> Phil and Carla have been married for two years, and Carla is now pregnant for the first time. Phil has had herpes for several years. They don't have sex when he's having an outbreak, and so far she seems not to have been infected. But what if she gets infected with herpes for the first time during pregnancy? This is a very high-risk situation, especially in the last trimester. What should they do?

> First, let's remember that most people who are infected with HSV-2 don't know it, and this might include Carla. Considering the fact of her exposure, she should be tested with a type-specific HSV serology to determine whether she truly is uninfected.

> If type-specific serology confirms that Carla is not infected with HSV-2, she and Phil should, at a minimum, refrain from all sexual activity during pregnancy when Phil is symptomatic, and should also use condoms for sex between outbreaks. In addition, Phil may choose to take antiviral medication suppressively to lower his rate of asymptomatic shedding and potentially reduce the likelihood of transmission. Then, too, there is always the option of abstaining from sex altogether, which would be a sensible precaution during the third trimester. Whatever precautions the couple chooses to take or not take, it's important that Carla's doctor or midwife be informed that Phil has herpes and she doesn't. It's also important to keep in mind that a substantial number of neonatal herpes cases are caused by HSV-1. So if Phil has a his-

tory of cold sores, avoiding oral-genital contact in late pregnancy should be considered.

When a woman has a first episode of herpes during pregnancy, timing is critical in the decision about vaginal delivery. If the episode occurs in the second half of her pregnancy, many experts recommend delivering the baby by C-section. One reason is that a substantial amount of asymptomatic shedding is likely in the few months immediately after a first episode. Another reason is that the body's immune response to herpes takes several months to become established, during which time neither mother nor baby has the protection of HSV antibodies.

WHEN NEWBORNS GET HERPES

Many babies are exposed to small amounts of HSV at birth yet resist infection, and all of the precautions outlined above are helpful in reducing the risk of infection. But some babies are infected with HSV at birth, and the consequences can often be severe. For infants, herpes is not just the possibility of an irritating rash. Because HSV can overpower the immature immune system, one in six babies with herpes dies, and survivors often suffer permanent brain damage.

Babies rarely show signs of herpes at birth. Neonatal infection—even in very serious cases—may cause no sores on the skin at all. Typically, however, herpes symptoms develop within several days to two weeks. These can include the classic herpes lesions seen in adults as well as jaundice, pneumonia, convulsions, general irritability, red swollen eyes (conjunctivitis), and lack of interest in food.

Because the initial symptoms of neonatal herpes infection overlap with those of more common childhood illnesses, diagnosis can be quite difficult. Viral culture is often used as a diagnostic test. Recently, a more sensitive DNA test called "polymerase chain reaction" (PCR) has been used to diagnose HSV infection and now is recommended in this setting.

The severity of herpes in newborns varies greatly. If infection is confined to the skin, eyes, and mouth, the infant's prognosis is usually good. But sometimes in newborns the virus can infect the blood and spread widely. In another frequent complication, herpes can attack the brain (encephalitis), causing irreversible damage.

With any form of neonatal infection, early diagnosis and treatment are critical. Acyclovir is effective in many cases. Some doctors will start an infant on acyclovir even before a herpes diagnosis is confirmed, provided there is strong suspicion that HSV is the cause of the child's illness. But this strategy is controversial in medical circles. Some doctors also will treat an infant if the mother was having a first episode of HSV infection during vaginal delivery, because the chances of transmission in this situation are so high.

PROTECTING THE BABY AT HOME

Even when a baby is born without herpes, it's important to remember there is still a risk of infection, and herpes can be a very serious illness in the first few weeks of life. Mothers and fathers with active herpes sores should take care to protect their babies. If you're having an outbreak (or even if you're not), some logical precautions include the following:

• Wash your hands before touching the baby.

• *If you have cold sores on your mouth,* wear a mask when you handle the baby to keep from inadvertently touching your mouth and then the baby.

• *If a visiting friend or relative has a cold sore,* warn him or her about the risks of spreading HSV to your newborn through a kiss or through careless touching and require him or her to wear a mask when handling the baby.

The point here is not to discourage all the touching and cuddling that go along with taking care of a newborn. That kind of contact is very necessary. But if you're having an outbreak, or a relative or friend is having an outbreak, safety is an important concern, and you'll want to take steps to protect your child.

WHAT YOU CAN DO

Many of the decisions about managing herpes at delivery call for discussion with your doctor or midwife. Be sure to tell your healthcare provider about your (or your partner's) history of genital herpes. Ask the provider to tell you about his or her standard procedures and the hospital's procedures regarding herpes, pregnancy, and delivery. Some of the questions you should ask are:

• How does your doctor or midwife determine the need for a C-section?

• Will he or she perform a thorough visual exam looking for signs of genital herpes early in labor?

• What types of monitors are routinely used? When might a fetal scalp monitor be used?

You also need to tell your obstetric healthcare provider if you plan to take (or have already taken) an antiviral drug during pregnancy. And of course, you'll want to tell your provider if you experience symptoms of herpes just prior to labor.

While it's smart to make plans in case you do have a herpes outbreak, keep in mind that the vast majority of women will not have an outbreak at delivery. And, as we've stressed, if you have a history of recurrent genital herpes, your baby already possesses antibodies to the virus. It's the babies born to mothers having a first episode during pregnancy who are at the highest risk of getting sick. Either way, the odds are in your favor.

15

THE BROADER SPECTRUM OF HSV INFECTION

In putting together this handbook, we've placed great emphasis on the fact that genital herpes is a very common infection that is certainly manageable—and for some people altogether trivial. We want people to keep herpes in this perspective.

You may, however, hear or read statements about herpes simplex that alarm you. Some may fall into the category of "herpes myths"—pure misinformation, such as the idea that people with herpes should never donate blood. Other statements, however, may prove to be accurate information that relates to *rare types* of HSV infection.

In reviewing what experts call the "full clinical spectrum" of HSV infection, we find a number of uncommon conditions that can result when either HSV-1 or HSV-2 breaks out of its usual pattern of latency and minor reactivations. In describing these conditions here, we run the risk of scaring you with what may sound like irrelevant information. If we were creating a book for drivers' education, this would be sort of like including a whole chapter on what to do if all four tires go flat at once. Nonetheless, we do want this book to serve as a useful information resource. We think it's important, therefore, to establish some basic facts about herpes complications, and to quash some of the misinformation currently spread.

HERPETIC WHITLOW

Among the forms of autoinoculation (self infection) already mentioned, herpetic whitlow, a herpes infection of the fingertip, deserves further explanation because it can occur in a number of ways. Generally, whitlow results when virus is spread to a finger that has a cut or abrasion. Once there, it can cause an outbreak with symptoms similar to those of oral-facial or genital herpes. Herpetic whitlow can also recur.

First, of course, the virus has to get to the finger. In people who have genital herpes, this is most likely to occur from touching your own lesions during a first episode (as was explained in Chapter 4). However, not all cases of whitlow result from genital herpes (HSV-2) infection. Some cases have been traced to adults who have an HSV-1 infection on the mouth or face and are in the habit of biting their fingernails. An active HSV-1 infection can deposit virus in saliva, and nail biting can create an opening in the skin that allows HSV a portal of entry.

In the past, herpetic whitlow afflicted significant numbers of dentists, surgeons, and other healthcare professionals whose hands were frequently in contact with patients' saliva. In recent years, however, the widespread use of latex gloves and other precautions appears to have reduced the incidence of whitlow among healthcare workers.

Today, most whitlow is caused by HSV-2 in sexually active

adults, almost always the result of hand contact with lesions during a first episode of genital herpes, prior to the development of a full immune response. Though the risk of herpetic whitlow is small in those with recurrent genital herpes, it's a good idea to avoid touching HSV lesions. If you do make contact, it's best to wash your hands right away. Soap and water will kill the virus and avert the risk of whitlow. And if you have oral-facial herpes, remember that biting your nails can be risky.

OCULAR HERPES

Ocular herpes, meaning HSV infection of the eye, is almost always caused by HSV-1 in adults and children. In newborn babies, it can be caused by HSV-2 acquired from the mother during birth. Ocular herpes usually occurs when latent HSV-1 from an earlier infection in the facial area reactivates and travels to the eye instead of the mouth or lips, but the eye can also be the site of a first infection. About 5% of people with an oral HSV-1 infection eventually develop ocular herpes.

Symptoms sometimes begin with blisters or cold sores on the eyelid and the itchy, watery sort of "pink eye" associated with conjunctivitis. Later symptoms typically include pain and sensitivity to light. Most cases will resolve on their own in two or three weeks, but when left untreated, ocular herpes can lead to painful lesions on the cornea.

More than 25% of people with ocular herpes experience recurrences. Repeated recurrences can result in corneal scarring, overgrowth of new blood vessels in the eye, and eventual blindness; however, a variety of effective topical and systemic treatments are available, including trifluridine, acyclovir, and vidarabine.

Whether or not vision is at risk depends on where in the eye the infection occurs, how often it recurs, and how quickly treatment is started.

HSV INFECTIONS OF THE NERVOUS SYSTEM

HSV can cause an infection of the nervous system called *meningitis*. Meningitis is an inflammation of the *meninges*, the protective membranes that cover the brain and spinal cord, and can be caused by a number of different infectious agents. When the cause is bacterial, the infection is called *septic meningitis*; when the cause is viral, it's called *aseptic meningitis*.

In children, the usual cause of HSV meningitis is HSV-1. In adults, most cases occur as a complication of a first infection with HSV-2. HSV meningitis is seen in more than 30% of women and about 10% of men experiencing a first HSV-2 infection. The principal symptoms include fever, stiff neck, intense headache, and aversion to bright light. Fortunately, HSV meningitis generally clears up by itself, recurs only infrequently, and causes no damage to the central nervous system. However, symptoms of numbness, tingling, muscle weakness, and difficult urination that are sometimes present with HSV meningitis may persist for a few months. Recurrence can be expected in 20% to 30% of cases, usually in association with a reactivation of genital herpes, but recurrent episodes of HSV meningitis tend to be milder than first episodes.

HSV is also linked to an extremely serious though extremely

rare infection called *encephalitis*, which is an infection of the brain tissue itself. In adults, HSV encephalitis is almost always caused by HSV-1. Most neonatal cases are caused by HSV-2. One reason it's so critical to prevent HSV-2 infection in newborns is that they are much more susceptible to encephalitis because of their immature immune system. (See Chapter 14 for more information on neonatal HSV infection and its prevention.)

Among adults, about half the cases of HSV encephalitis are first infections of HSV-1; the rest occur as a complication of recurrent infection; but in either case, course and outcome are the same. HSV encephalitis is marked initially by fever, headache, and confusion, but patients rapidly suffer more serious effects such as seizure and delirium. Only about 1,000 cases are seen each year in the U.S., but without antiviral therapy, 70% of those afflicted will die. Survivors may suffer permanent brain damage.

DISSEMINATED HSV INFECTION AND HSV INFECTION IN THE IMMUNOCOMPROMISED

Viremia refers to the finding of virus in the bloodstream. Viremia is probably present to some extent in every case of primary (first) infection with HSV, but in otherwise healthy individuals with normal immune function, it's usually not a problem. It is possible, however, for HSV in the bloodstream to cause a widespread HSV infection called a *disseminated* infection, which may cause extensive lesions on the skin and affect internal organs as well. (Even in cases that appear to be limited to the skin, some internal lesions are likely.) Disseminated HSV infection is a serious condition that requires immediate medical attention and antiviral therapy. A number of organs may be involved, but the liver is the focus of greatest concern.

Those most susceptible to disseminated HSV infection are people whose immune systems are suppressed (or *compromised*). Immunocompromise can occur naturally as a congenital defect, or it can be induced by malnutrition, severe burn injury, diseases such as HIV/AIDS and cancer, radical medical interventions such as radiation therapy, or immunosuppressive drugs used to prevent rejection of transplanted organs and tissues.

People with suppressed immune systems are sometimes vulnerable to complications if they have either genital or oral-facial HSV. Some with recurrent genital herpes have lengthy outbreaks that must be treated with antiviral medication. People with AIDS, in particular, may have severe and lengthy outbreaks. In fact, HSV is one of the so-called *opportunistic infections* that define a patient's transition from being merely HIV positive to having AIDS.

Acyclovir, valacyclovir, and famciclovir are often used to treat HSV infection in AIDS patients. Episodic or suppressive therapeutic strategies may be followed, but in either case, the patient often receives doses higher than those given to patients with normal immune function. But even at higher doses, first-line antiviral therapy may fail to control the infection.

While the interaction between HSV and HIV has many facets, a major reason for treatment failure is the emergence of virus that is resistant or less sensitive to acyclovir or penciclovir. Naturally occurring resistant strains of HSV are found in about 1% of people with normal immune function, but even so, these strains are of no known clinical significance, as most patients respond to antiviral therapy regardless of the presence of resistant strains. In immunocompromised patients, however, HSV (including resistant strains) is present in much greater volume. Antiviral therapy knocks out the susceptible strains, but the patient's lack of natural defenses and the presence of an unusually large amount of resistant virus can lead to the overgrowth of resistant virus and a persistent infection that is immune to first-line antiviral therapy. In these cases, medications such as intravenous foscarnet or the topical drugs cidofovir and trifluridine, which have a different way of attacking HSV, are sometimes used.

The emergence of resistant strains of bacteria due to the overuse and misuse of antibiotics has become a very real problem, especially in the hospital setting. Clinicians have naturally been concerned that the widespread use of acyclovir might also lead to the emergence of resistant HSV, which could be problematic for the general immunocompetent population. But so far, no evidence has been found to suggest that this concern is warranted.

HSV INFECTION AND BLOOD DONATION

ASHA has occasionally fielded questions and comments from people who have been deferred from donating blood because they had a recurring herpes infection or because they were on daily suppressive antiviral therapy. However, according to a medical representative at the national office of the American Red Cross, neither daily antiviral therapy nor recurrent HSV infection itself are legitimate grounds for deferral, and the latter applies to infection with HSV-1 or HSV-2. The policy, as expressed by the national office, recognizes that HSV "lives" in the nervous system, not in the blood, and there is no documented case of HSV transmission via blood infusion. However, it is clear that local chapters of the Red Cross may have different rules and regulations and that the people conducting the screening exams may have different understandings of the national policy.

As noted earlier in this chapter, some degree of HSV viremia (HSV in the bloodstream) is probably present in the majority of first infections. While this HSV viremia is of no known relevance when it comes to blood donation, it is advisable to abstain from blood donation during a first episode of HSV infection. Aside from the fact that you probably have at least some small amount of HSV in your bloodstream, it's also true that you're unwell just now. Chances are if you are in the midst of a true first HSV infection, donating blood is the last thing you'll feel like doing, and it just doesn't make sense to further weaken yourself by giving blood. In fact, donating blood is not recommended for persons with flu or any other acute illness. And even though there are no official blood-donation restrictions for persons subject to recurrent HSV infection, if you are having a recurrence and feeling sick with the symptoms, it makes more sense to wait until the current outbreak subsides.

THE BOTTOM LINE

If you have genital herpes, take precautions to avoid the problems of autoinoculation. If you experience a first episode of HSV infection, try to avoid touching the lesions, and wash your hands immediately afterward if you do touch them. This simple step can help you avoid herpetic whitlow. Also, remember to keep your hands away from your eyes when HSV is active. Most cases of ocular herpes in adults are due to HSV-1, but it is possible to transfer HSV-2 by hand from genital lesions to your eyes.

Remember that complications such as disseminated HSV infection are most likely to appear in people with compromised immune systems. If you have a history of herpes infection and are to undergo cancer treatment (or any other procedure or intervention) that could suppress your immune function, tell your doctor about your medical history so prophylactic antiviral therapy can be considered. The same advice goes for people who are newly diagnosed with HIV: tell your doctor if you have a history of herpes infection. You may benefit from suppressive antiviral therapy.

16

DIAGNOSTIC
TESTS

⟨◎⟩

"Two years ago I had some sores on my labia and went to the doctor," says a caller to the National Herpes Hotline. "He just looked at them and told me I had herpes. Then he gave me a prescription and said I might have more trouble later on. Well, I haven't had any symptoms in all this time, and I'm wondering: Maybe this isn't herpes. Could it be something else?"

Herpes simplex is the most common cause of genital sores or ulcers in the United States, and often it can be recognized by the trained eye of a medical professional. However, HSV can be confused with other infections, and some people have good reason to question the diagnosis they received. In one recent study, the rate of false positive diagnosis was 20%, and some studies have pointed to an even greater likelihood of false negatives—meaning that herpes is more often underdiagnosed. Consequently, we recommend that everyone who visits a doctor for treatment of herpes request a laboratory test; this can confirm a diagnosis that may have been based on visual clues or the patient's medical history.

VIRAL CULTURE

There are several diagnostic tests currently available, and more reach the market each year. At present, the test used most often to diagnose herpes is called *viral culture*. Using a swab, the healthcare provider gathers infected cells from an active herpes lesion. The swab is then placed into a special solution and sent to a laboratory. At the lab, virus from the swab is allowed to grow for several days in a collection of healthy cells. If HSV is indeed present on the swab, it will cause certain changes in the cell culture that can be seen easily under a microscope. In essence, viral culture transplants the virus into another setting and allows it to grow until its effects on cells are visible. Then the cells are stained with a specific antibody that will react with one or both HSV types to confirm that the virus is herpes simplex.

The major advantage of viral culture is its *specificity*, meaning it will not be positive for herpes simplex virus if another infection is causing the cell changes.

Though viral culture is the most widely used laboratory test for HSV, it does have drawbacks and limitations. Samples for viral culture must be taken when and where virus can be found, either from lesions on the surface of the skin or from mucous membranes on internal surfaces, such as those of the cervix. The best samples come from lesions that contain large amounts of virus and have not yet had a chance to form a crust or scab. If the target lesion is in the process of healing, viral culture often yields a false negative result: the swab doesn't pick up enough live virus, and the test fails to find HSV, even though herpes really is the culprit. Viral culture is most likely to be positive (80% to 90% of the time) during first episodes, when large amounts of virus are present. During recurrent episodes, the likelihood of a positive is between 30% and 60%. In technical terms, then, while culture has good specificity, it is not highly *sensitive.*

Another potential disadvantage of viral culture is that it often takes many hours before cellular changes occur in the culture medium, so the results are anything but rapid. Most lab reports take from two to seven days for completion, and waiting for the results may test your patience. Though clearly not infallible, viral culture remains the most widely used, and perhaps most reliable, tool for an initial herpes diagnosis, if lesions are present.

Viral culture costs anywhere from $40 to $100 (depending on the lab chosen and not including the cost of an office visit). If the results are negative and your healthcare provider has good reason to suspect HSV anyway, you should arrange to come back to the office promptly the next time you have an outbreak so a better sample can be obtained.

TYPE 1 OR TYPE 2?

As we've already said, it's useful to know whether your herpes symptoms are caused by HSV-1 or HSV-2, the major reason being that genital HSV-1 infection is less likely to cause frequent recurrent outbreaks. If you're in the midst of a first episode, you might find it reassuring to know you're dealing with the less troublesome of the two viral types. Determining viral type can be done in a number of ways. Most commonly, lab technicians take an HSV sample grown in cell culture—a proven HSV specimen—and expose it to type-specific antibodies. As mentioned above, viral typing is often a routine step for confirming the cell changes in HSV cultures, entailing no additional costs.

SEROLOGY

One of the disadvantages of all the viral culture methods and the confirmatory tests described above is that they only work well when herpes is in its active phase and genital sores are present. But what about the person who has had only one outbreak and now questions the diagnosis? What about all the people who have mild symptoms that test negative in a viral culture, or those whose partners develop herpes and claim they have not been unfaithful? Perhaps more important, what about all the people who are infected with HSV but are unaware of it?

One diagnostic tool that skirts the problem of sampling active lesions is a blood test called a *serologic assay* or, more simply, a *serology*. HSV serologic assays detect antibodies to HSV that are made by your body as a natural defensive response to infection. Immune response varies from one individual to the next, so it's difficult to say exactly how long it may take for detectable antibodies to form. However, beginning just a few days after initial infection with HSV, antibodies are produced in growing numbers, and within a few weeks to a few months, they can be detected whether HSV is in an active or latent phase. Their presence certifies infection. Thus, serologic tests are a standard method of diagnosing a number of infections that a person may have acquired in the past. For example, the standard HIV test is a serologic test for antibodies to HIV.

A serologic assay can be a powerful diagnostic tool, but only if it can tell the difference between HSV-1 and HSV-2 infections. Here's the problem: an estimated 66% of adults in the U.S. are infected with HSV-1 (the "cold sore" virus, usually acquired in childhood). If the serology used is not *type-specific* (that is, able to distinguish HSV-1 antibodies from HSV-2 antibodies), a positive result really tells us nothing about the likelihood of genital herpes. The test may just be detecting an earlier oral HSV-1 infection and is, therefore, effectively worthless. Unfortunately, many serologies claim to be type-specific, and their lab reports show separate readings for HSV-1 and HSV-2, but most of these tests will cross-react with antibodies for either viral type (and sometimes with other herpesviruses). What shows up as HSV-2 may really be HSV-1 and vice versa. In fact, many experts believe these nonspecific serologic tests should be taken off the market or clearly labeled as unable to distinguish between antibodies to HSV-1 and HSV-2.

Does this mean it's best to write off serologies altogether? No. Bona fide tests that are truly type-specific are available. With these, patients can know for certain what researchers call their *serostatus*—that is, do they have HSV-1, HSV-2, neither, or both? And patients can know this whether they have symptomatic outbreaks or not. These type-specific tests have proved extremely valuable in research to determine the extent of herpes infection among adults and in the study of patterns of viral shedding and other aspects of how HSV behaves in the body. In a wide range of research studies, type-specific serology is a valuable tool for understanding the intricacies of HSV.

Serologic testing has changed rapidly in recent years and is no longer confined to the research setting. As of this writing there are two diagnostic companies offering commercially available tests with proven accuracy in determining HSV viral type from a blood sample. They include Diagnology, which produces the POCkit HSV-2 Rapid Test; and Focus Technologies, which offers two different HSV tests (see Table). Kits by other manufacturers may join these in the commercial market, pending FDA approval.

Commercially Available Type-Specific Serologic Tests for HSV Antibody

Test Name	Company	Sensitivity[1]	Specificity[2]	Comments
HerpeSelect™ 1 & 2 ELISA	Focus Technologies	96–100	97–100	Collection through standard blood draw. Results in 1 to 2 weeks.
HerpeSelect™ 1 & 2 Immunoblot	Focus Technologies	97–100	98	Collection through standard blood draw. Results in 1 to 2 weeks.
POCkit™ HSV-2 Rapid Test	Diagnology	93–100	94–97	Collection through finger prick. Results in < 10 minutes. Standard blood draw also available.

Table reflects FDA-approved tests widely available as of January 2002. Range of scores reflects results from several studies using various standards of comparison.

1 – Sensitivity refers to a test's ability to detect the presence of antibodies whenever they are present. A sensitive test avoids false negatives.

2 – Specificity refers to a test's reliability in showing a positive result *only* when antibodies are present. A specific test avoids false positives.

Source: Data adapted from Ashley RL, Sorting out the new HSV type-specific tests. Sex Trans Infect 2001; 77:232-237.

The "gold standard" of HSV serologic testing is the Western blot, developed by academic research labs such as the Virology Laboratory at the University of Washington in Seattle. This test has been used in many research studies and has been available by request to private practitioners around the United States.

Each of these tests uses a slightly different methodology, and costs may vary substantially from one to another. The least time-consuming is the POCkit HSV-2 Rapid Test, which can be done with a serum sample from a finger prick. Assuming the provider has the proper lab facilities, results are available in less than 10 minutes. The other tests listed above require a standard blood draw, which is then sent off to a specialized laboratory for testing. Results for these generally take one to two weeks.

Some individuals infected with HSV-2 will develop antibodies that can be detected by these type-specific tests within two weeks, but most will not. For this reason, experts usually recommend that patients wait 12 to 16 weeks after exposure to HSV before seeking a serologic test.

As valuable as type-specific serology has proved to be, there are practical limits to its usefulness. It's important that you understand exactly what a serologic result means:

> • If your serologic test is positive for HSV-2, we know that you have been infected with HSV-2 at some time in the past (but we don't know when). It is highly likely that your HSV-2 infection is a genital infection for the simple

reason that almost all HSV-2 infections are genital. This is true even if you've never experienced any genital symptoms.

• If your serology is positive for HSV-1, we know that you have been infected with HSV-1 at some time in your life, and while it is probably an oral or facial infection (even if you have no history of cold sores), you should be aware that a growing number of genital herpes infections are caused by HSV-1.

• If your test result is negative for HSV-1 and HSV-2, you're not out of the woods just yet. Remember, type-specific serologies detect antibodies to HSV and are of limited value during and immediately after a first episode of infection, because you may not have had adequate time to form antibodies to the virus.

Type-specific serology can be of tremendous value in a number of settings. Remember Phil and Carla, the expectant parents in Chapter 14? Phil knew he had an HSV-2 infection; Carla's serostatus was unknown but presumed to be negative. If it truly were the case that Carla had never been infected with HSV-1 or HSV-2 and thus had no antibodies to either virus, an accurate type-specific serology could alert Carla's obstetric caregivers to a potentially serious complication: namely, that of Carla's acquiring a first HSV infection late in her pregnancy, a dangerous circumstance for the fetus.

Type-specific serology is also valuable in cases where a patient has reason to question a herpes diagnosis that was never confirmed by laboratory test. Take the case of Larry, who was given a visual diagnosis of herpes years ago but whose viral culture always came back negative. He has only the mildest rash in the genital area about once a year. Is this really herpes? Taken together with his history, a serology positive for HSV-2 is strong evidence that the answer is yes.

Type-specific serology can also simplify a couple's sex life and relieve the stress and apprehension of HSV transmission. Imagine a case in which one partner in the couple (let's call them Cathy and Mike) has a confirmed HSV-2 infection, and the other partner's serostatus is unknown. Cathy knows she has genital herpes, and Mike *thinks* he does not. (But of course most who have herpes don't know they have it.) Mike could undergo a type-specific serologic test, and if the result came back positive for HSV-2, the couple could quit worrying about Mike acquiring genital herpes from Cathy. They might then choose to forego the precaution of condoms, if fear of HSV transmission were their only reason for using condoms.

As this technology hits the market, the biggest problem for patients and healthcare providers alike may be distinguishing the quality tests from the impostors. Guidelines published by the American Medical Association and by the U.S. Centers for Disease Control are intended to help medical professionals sort through the conflicting claims of diagnostic companies and identify the truly accurate serologic tests. Consumers wishing to get more information can contact the National Herpes Hotline for details about these products and possible updates. (See Resource List on page 221 for Web site and telephone listings for the diagnostic tests mentioned above.)

In addition to possible confusion over which tests are the most accurate, there is also some disagreement among medical experts as to the best uses for type-specific blood tests. In which situations should they be employed? Can they be relied upon for diagnosing a person with an apparent first episode? Will they have value in testing someone who has a history of unexplained genital symptoms? Should they be used in testing all persons at risk for herpes?

While these and other questions are currently under discussion, there is emerging consensus that type-specific serologic tests will be very helpful in two clinical situations:

- *History of recurrent genital symptoms:* In many cases, patients present to a healthcare provider seeking diagnosis of genital symptoms that recur from time to time but are not present at the time of the clinic visit. When the patient's history (including risk factors and description of symptoms) suggests the possibility of herpes, a serologic test can provide very useful information. Specifically, a test result positive for HSV-2 would be a very strong indication that herpes had been causing the symptoms.

- *Discordant couples:* If one partner has been diagnosed with herpes and the couple is faced with decisions about how to prevent the spread of genital herpes, the first question demanding an answer might be this: Does the second partner already have herpes anyway? As we showed in the early chapters of this book, it's quite common for an individual to have herpes and not know it. Testing may provide the information that both partners already have the same serotype, and this would mean they faced little or no risk of transmission anyway. For example, if Jack has been diagnosed with HSV-2 genital herpes, and Jill's test shows that she also has HSV-2 antibodies, many of the precautions a couple might take may be seen as unnecessary.

In addition to these two scenarios, some are advocating type-specific tests for two other situations:

• *STD screening:* Many people have reason to seek a medical check-up to find out whether they are free of sexually transmitted diseases. Perhaps, for example, they have a relatively new partner, have initially used condoms as a precaution, and now are reconsidering the question of whether any form of safer sex is really necessary. A visit to the healthcare provider, they reason, will enable a thorough check for STDs.

First of all, it should be mentioned that there is a wide range of practices when it comes to STD testing, and even some common infections such as chlamydia may not be part of a clinic's routine testing. And before the advent of commercial serologic tests for HSV, there was really no practical way of testing for herpes unless genital lesions were present. Now that serologic tests are widely available, the question becomes: should these tests be more widely used? Experts take a variety of positions on this, but a growing number support the idea that a person requesting to be "checked for STDs" should be offered an HSV serologic test—or, at the very least, should be informed (if the test is not routinely available) that they are *not* being tested for herpes when they request their STD checkup.

• *Routine Screening of Pregnant Women:* As we explained in Chapter 14, the risk of neonatal herpes is highest when a pregnant woman acquires genital herpes during pregnancy. The role of serologic testing, then, would be to identify women who are free of HSV infection—who are at risk for either HSV-1 or HSV-2. Once identified, these seronegative women could be made aware of the risk of acquiring herpes from a sexual partner and could be educated about prevention measures such as use of condoms or abstaining from sex in the third trimester. A number of experts in this area have suggested a model in which serologic tests can also be offered to the partners of seronegative women, to determine whether a risk of transmission exists within that particular couple.

The notion of routine blood testing for women in pregnancy poses a number of challenges, and as of this writing there are no published guidelines for the use of such an approach.

OTHER COMMON DIAGNOSTIC TOOLS

Among the alternatives to the viral culture is a test that identifies HSV antigens, which are virus particles that provoke the immune system to respond. This procedure begins the same way a virus culture does: the doctor uses a swab to retrieve virus from an active lesion, and the lab then combines this sample with HSV antibodies and a detector system. Detector systems can be enzymes that cause color changes or fluorescence if HSV antigens are present in the specimen.

Because antigen test kits don't require HSV to replicate and grow, this test is faster than viral culture, taking only a few hours (though results will seldom be reported back from the lab this quickly). The test also rates well in the area of specificity, rarely confusing HSV with something else. Some antigen tests are equal to or better than viral culture in sensitivity when the specimen is taken from lesions. And the cost of antigen testing is generally in the same range as the cell culture, though prices fluctuate from lab to lab. However, these tests in general cannot tell whether the infection is caused by HSV-1 or HSV-2.

Other testing methods sometimes used to diagnose herpes include the Tzanck test and Pap smear to identify HSV-infected cells. A physician scrapes herpes lesions and may treat the sample with various stains. When the samples are examined under a microscope, certain telltale signs of herpes infection can be spotted by the trained eye. These procedures are rapid and simple, but they require a "judgment call" by the lab technician. Under a microscope, changes caused by other herpesviruses may look very similar to those caused by HSV, so both tests leave lots of room for human error.

An additional word about Pap smears is in order. Many women believe that their annual or biannual Pap test looks for a number of STDs and that a normal result indicates the absence of STDs. Unfortunately, this is not true. Pap smears check for abnormal cells in cervical tissue, and by proxy, often detect an STD called human papillomavirus. But a Pap smear is not a specific test for any STD and is not used to look for HSV.

However, occasionally a Pap smear will detect cell changes that look like those caused by HSV.

Lastly, a type of test you may begin hearing more about is *polymerase chain reaction*, or PCR. As with culture, this test detects virus that has reactivated and traveled from the nerves to the skin—genital skin, for example. More sensitive than any of the technologies listed here, PCR may one day offer a very rapid, extremely sensitive, type-specific diagnostic test for HSV. It's currently used for clinical diagnosis by many of the country's top university laboratories, and some commercial laboratories now have it on the market. In particular, PCR has become the test of choice for herpes infections of the central nervous system (meningitis and encephalitis) and HSV infection in newborns. As yet, however, there is no scientific consensus on the general use of PCR in diagnosing genital herpes infections.

17

NEW RESEARCH, NEW HOPE

Living in a world of rapid scientific and technological change, we'd like to think that any day now modern medicine will find a way to wipe out genital herpes instead of just holding it in check. But the truth is, we're unlikely to see a real cure any time soon.

The great difficulty in developing a cure lies in the dual nature of herpes simplex virus infection — it has active *and* latent phases. Today's antiviral drugs (acyclovir, valacyclovir, and famciclovir) are very effective against *active* virus, such as HSV replicating in the skin. In fact, these antivirals are effectively "switched on" by an enzyme that is produced only when HSV is replicating (active). But today's antivirals do nothing to combat dormant HSV, because dormant HSV doesn't put out the requisite chemical signals.

Further complicating the challenge is that any drug developed to root out latent HSV infection must locate and eliminate dormant virus without killing the nerve cells (ganglia) in which it resides. Nerve tissue poses an especially tricky problem because it doesn't regenerate; kill too many nerve cells, and the cure is worse than the disease.

Does all this mean there's no hope? Has medical science given up? No—not by a long shot. Promising avenues of HSV research include the following:

1. *Refining our understanding of existing antivirals* — Can they be used to prevent or reduce the transmission of HSV?

2. *Developing HSV vaccines, both prophylactic (preventative) and therapeutic* — When we hear the word 'vaccine' we tend to think in terms of disease prevention, but vaccines can also be used therapeutically to modify an established infection. How close are we to perfecting either approach?

3. *Developing new drugs with different modes of action* — Can we attack HSV in ways different from the approaches used in our existing antivirals? Can we boost the immune system to fight the infection better?

ONGOING HSV TRANSMISSION STUDY

One of the significant challenges of genital herpes, both at a personal level and from a public health standpoint, is preventing the spread of the infection. This is complicated by the fact that so many people with genital HSV do not recognize their symptoms, and by the fact that the infection can be spread when no obvious signs or symptoms are present. By now, it's well known that antiviral drugs reduce the frequency of recurrent symptomatic herpes infection and also reduce asymptomatic shedding. Given these two factors, do antivirals also reduce the risk of transmission? It seems plausible that they do. But any such assertion requires sound medical research. To that end,

GlaxoSmithKline is presently conducting a study among 1,500 monogamous, heterosexual, discordant couples (couples in which one person has genital herpes and the other does not) to determine if the antiviral valacyclovir can reduce or prevent the transmission of genital herpes. Preliminary results from this study may be available late in 2002.

VACCINE RESEARCH AND DEVELOPMENT

Just about everyone in this country has some experience with vaccination. Tens of millions of Americans have a small round scar on their upper arm where they were vaccinated for smallpox during childhood. Most of us have been vaccinated for polio, tetanus, and a host of other infectious diseases.

Vaccination introduces a foreign substance (an antigen) into our bodies in a controlled manner, so our immune system has a chance to prepare a response to the antigen. This response includes the body's production of antibodies as well as the cellular immune response described in Chapter 4. Both of these internal defense systems fight off infection when we are exposed to disease-causing bacteria and viruses. The idea is that vaccination will cause production of sufficient antibodies, or a sufficiently strong cellular immune response, to ward off future infection.

One major divide in the field of vaccine development centers on whether a vaccine is designed to prevent infection from occurring in the first place or whether it's designed to prevent or lessen the symptoms of an infection. In a *prophylactic* application, a vaccine prevents infection. In a *therapeutic* application, a vaccine alters only the symptoms and course of infection. With regard to HSV infection, researchers are exploring both ways to use vaccines: prophylactically, to prevent HSV-2 infection from becoming established; and therapeutically, to prevent or decrease the frequency of symptoms once it's already established.

THE HSV SUBUNIT VACCINE

An HSV-2 subunit vaccine is made using just a portion (subunit) of the HSV particle to trigger an immune response, rather than using the whole virus. Two companies have undertaken the development of an HSV subunit vaccine. One, Chiron, has discontinued work on its vaccine, having found it ineffective in clinical trials. The other company, GlaxoSmithKline, has had some success.*

As of this writing, results are available from the first round of Phase 3 trials of the GSK HSV-2 subunit vaccine— two double-blind, placebo-controlled studies. Both studies were carried out in *discordant couples*, meaning that one person had genital herpes and one did not. Study participants in the category of *uninfected* tested negative for HSV-2, and the study included some who had not been infected with either HSV-1 or HSV-2.

Interestingly, the GSK study assessed effectiveness in two very different ways. First, the study followed all uninfected subjects closely to see whether they developed any signs or symptoms of disease. Secondly, uninfected partners in the study were tested at

---

*Author's Note: SmithKline Beecham (SKB) merged with Glaxo Wellcome in December of 2000 to form GlaxoSmithKline (GSK).

intervals to see whether they had *seroconverted*, that is, acquired infection as evidenced by the presence of circulating antibodies to HSV-2.

In the end, the GSK subunit vaccine performed very differently depending on the measure used—and perhaps most important, depending on the segment of the uninfected population studied. Bottom line: The vaccine proved successful only in women who had not previously been infected with HSV-1. In the two studies, 48% and 39% of this subpopulation did not become infected with HSV-2 during the 19 months of the study, while 73% and 74% of this subpopulation did not develop symptoms.

Why the apparent protective effect only in women without prior HSV-1? Some researchers believe HSV-1 and HSV-2 are so closely related that infection with one viral type usually gives a person partial immunity to the other type. By this logic, women with prior HSV-1 already carry substantial immunity—immunity which the vaccine could not improve upon. There are conflicting data on this question of partial immunity, and the reasons why the GSK subunit vaccine proved effective only in *women* without prior HSV-1 infection remains to be clarified.

At the end of the day, vaccine research has been boosted by the fact that the subunit vaccine holds some promise of preventing or suppressing severe primary episodes of genital herpes in one subpopulation. Questions remain, however, about whether this vaccine has any effect on asymptomatic viral shedding. It's possible that those who acquire HSV-2 after vaccination might be free of symptoms but still have infectious asymptomatic periods—an important public health issue. Further research is under way.

THE DISC HSV VACCINE

A British pharmaceutical company (Cantab) has developed a novel approach to HSV vaccination with a proprietary technology they call *disabled infectious single cycle virus* or DISC. Unlike the subunit vaccine, which uses just a portion of the virus to trigger an immune response, the DISC vaccine uses whole, live, genetically disabled HSV-2 virus. The disabled HSV-2 can enter cells and trigger an immune response, but because it cannot go through more than one cycle of replication, it is incapable of establishing full-blown HSV-2 infection. Developers hope that using whole, live virus will produce a broader immune response than a viral subunit. Early clinical studies are reported to have shown good safety and tolerability for the DISC approach, and more data are awaited. We do not know yet whether this vaccine will decrease the number of recurrences in people with genital herpes. Trials of this product as a prophylactic vaccine have not been started as of this writing. The process has been complicated by the merger of Glaxo Wellcome (which has licensed the DISC vaccine) with SmithKline Beecham (developer of the subunit vaccine) in December of 2000. To prevent anticompetitive dominance of the vaccine market, the U.S. Federal Trade Commission required the new company—GlaxoSmithKline—to stop work on DISC as a prophylactic vaccine, but work on its therapeutic potential continues.

RESIQUIMOD

Pharmaceutical developers are also conducting trials with *resiquimod*, which belongs to a new class of drug called immune modulators. Administered topically, resiquimod is designed to work by stimulating a strong local immune response that would in turn boost the cellular immune response to HSV. In a randomized, double-blind, placebo-controlled trial, 52 people with frequently recurring genital herpes (6 or more recurrences/year) were treated with varying strengths of resiquimod gel or a placebo gel while having recurrent symptoms. The patients were treated once or twice weekly for 3 weeks and observed for 6 months. At the end of 6 months, 32% of the resiquimod group had no recurrences of genital herpes, while only 6% of the placebo group remained free of recurrent disease. Among patients in whom genital herpes recurred, resiquimod-treated patients had a longer average interval to first recurrence than the placebo group (169 days vs. 57 days).

As of this writing, a Phase III study is testing the compound in a larger group of patients. It is hoped that repeated applications of resiquimod will help patients with recurrent genital herpes by keeping them symptom-free for long periods of time. Its effect on asymptomatic shedding will also be studied. If successful, it may prove to be the first topical treatment able to significantly benefit genital herpes patients.

OTHER APPROACHES

But what, you may ask, about a *real cure*? What about something that doesn't just slow down HSV? Where is the medical innovation that would help people who already have herpes—not just the uninfected? Every month the American Social Health Association gets scores of inquiries like these. Some come from people who are recently diagnosed and have trouble accepting that medical science doesn't have more to offer. Some come in response to news reports about novel compounds that show promise against one virus or another. Others simply reflect the view that more research is needed and that HSV is probably low on the list of national priorities.

There are, in fact, a large number of researchers investigating completely new approaches to HSV, including chemical compounds that may one day prove useful in new medications. In addition, some scientists are trying to unravel the mystery of what is loosely called HSV's "on-off switch." That is, there may be a specific gene that determines whether HSV is latent or active, and science may one day be able to keep this "switch" turned permanently off.

The thing to keep in mind if you see a news clip heralding a revolutionary breakthrough is that the process of bringing a new drug to market is long, expensive, and complex. Test-tube experiments are followed by laboratory tests on animals, which are then followed by exhaustive tests or "clinical trials" in humans. These trials—organized in three separate phases—focus first on safety, and later on both the safety and effectiveness of the drug in question.

The U.S. Pharmaceutical Manufacturers Association claims that only 1 in 5,000 new chemicals investigated by the industry ever makes it to the drugstore. It also estimates that the average new drug takes 12–15 years and approximately $500 million to bring to market. Other experts say the average cost is far lower. Either way, the path is full of pitfalls, and there are a myriad of would-be miracle drugs left by the wayside every year.

While herpes is not public health priority "number one" these days, it's worth mentioning that a major herpes breakthrough of any kind is potentially worth a lot of money. For example, with millions of symptomatic herpes patients in the United States alone, any treatment or diagnostic test has the potential for major commercial success.

The point is that herpes is not a lost and forgotten infection in the realm of biomedical research. If you have herpes, and you're anxious to hear about important scientific advances, there are any number of medical journals and texts that report on new developments. Many of these are summarized for lay audiences in *the helper*, a quarterly journal of the American Social Health Association. (See the Resource List on page 221 for details.)

18

OTHER SEXUALLY
TRANSMITTED DISEASES

⟨◎⟩

Although herpes is the principal subject of our book, it's just one component of a broader epidemic of sexually transmitted disease in this country. The American Social Health Association estimates there were 15.3 million new cases of sexually transmitted infection (including herpes) in the U.S. in 1996—the last year for which comprehensive estimates have been completed. While some of these STDs are bacterial infections and easily cured, others are lifelong viral infections for which no cure presently exists. And while some are becoming less common (or in some cases, merely less talked about), others are on the rise. When you're discussing issues of sexual health with a current or prospective sex partner, both of you should be considering the broader spectrum of sexually transmitted infection. Women *especially* need to protect themselves from STDs because of the associated increased risks of reproductive problems and injury to the newborn.

Note on terminology: When we discuss the presence of disease in a specific community or in the general population, we use the terms *incidence* and *prevalence*. Prevalence is how many people in the population have a given disease at any given time. Incidence is the number of *new cases* occurring in a certain time period. For example, we believe that at least 45 million people in the U.S. are currently infected with herpes; that's our number for prevalence. We expect at least 1 million new cases to be added to that number each year, so 1 million is the annual incidence. In the summaries of other STDs that follow, we will be talking about annual incidence (the number of new cases per year) unless otherwise noted.

CHLAMYDIA — A bacterium, *Chlamydia trachomatis* infects an estimated 3 million people in the U.S. each year. Antibiotics can rid the body of chlamydia in a matter of days, but people with chlamydia often fail to get prompt treatment because they have no idea they're infected. The reason is that chlamydia causes no signs or symptoms of illness in up to 50% of men and 75% of women. When symptoms are present, they often include painful urination for men and vaginal discharge for women. Unfortunately, the scarcity of obvious symptoms doesn't mean chlamydia is harmless. Left untreated, it can cause a variety of reproductive problems. In women, it can lead to pelvic inflammatory disease (PID) and tubal scarring, resulting in other damage and ectopic pregnancy. *Chlamydia is so common that if you're sexually active, with multiple partners, the U.S. Centers for Disease Control and Prevention (CDC) strongly recommends you have a screening test at least once a year. All sexually active women under 20 years of age should also be tested annually.*

GONORRHEA — You might think of gonorrhea as a sort of dinosaur STD, one that was a problem decades ago but has since been brought under control. Not so. While the annual incidence (the number of new cases per year) has been declining, ASHA estimates there were still around 650,000 new cases in 1996. The rate of infection is especially high among teenagers and minorities. The symptoms are similar to those of chlamydia, and people who are infected, especially women, can be completely without symptoms. Most cases are easily cured with antibiotics. But as with chlamydia, left untreated, gonorrhea can lead to reproductive tract infections associated with pelvic inflammatory disease, ectopic pregnancy, and infertility.

SYPHILIS — Public health officials have been making a concerted effort to eliminate syphilis in the U.S. and have had much success. The CDC estimates there were fewer than 6,000 cases of primary or secondary syphilis in the year 2000—down 30% from 1997 figures. Running a complicated course once inside the human body, syphilis first causes noticeable ulcers on the genitals, which in some cases may resemble herpes lesions. Untreated, syphilis will seem to disappear spontaneously, but the disease actually goes into a latent phase that can be followed by increasingly serious health complications and death. The complications include problems with the central nervous system or with the heart and blood vessels. The good news: once diagnosed, syphilis is usually easily cured with antibiotics.

HUMAN PAPILLOMAVIRUS (HPV) — Considered uncommon until the past 10 years, genital HPV is now detected by more sophisticated tests in a surprising percentage of adults. It is the single most common STD in the United States. The 1996

ASHA estimate of the number of new cases was 5.5 million (incidence). Prevalence nationwide is estimated at 20 million There are many different types of human papillomavirus. Some cause genital warts of various shapes and sizes; others cause changes in the cells of the cervix that predispose infected women to cervical cancer. It usually is HPV, then, that causes abnormal Pap smear results.

The signs and symptoms of HPV infection are diverse, ranging from nothing at all to fleshy, cauliflower-like warts. Also like herpes, HPV can defy treatment and persist for years, though there's also evidence that the immune system sometimes clears the virus over time. There are several different treatments that remove the warts themselves or remove the affected tissue on the cervix, but treatment isn't certain to eradicate the virus, and genital warts often recur after treatment.

Among the types of HPV linked to cervical infection, some are considered especially "high risk"—meaning more likely to cause a form of cervical precancer requiring treatment. A new diagnostic test can be run on a Pap smear specimen to determine if high-risk HPV types are present, but there is still debate in the medical community about whether such tests should be used routinely.

HEPATITIS B & C — Infection by the hepatitis B virus (HBV) is the most common sexually transmitted form of hepatitis (liver infection). About two-thirds of all HBV infections are spread sexually through body fluids such as blood, semen, or vaginal fluids. People who contract HBV can develop chronic liver disease entailing liver cell damage, cirrhosis, and increased risk for liver cancer. ASHA estimates about 77,000 new sexually transmitted cases a year (incidence) and a total number of sexually transmitted cases (prevalence) of 750,000. HBV infection cannot be cured, but there is a vaccine that can prevent it. The CDC recommends vaccination for all infants, adolescents, and sexually active adults.

Infection with hepatitis C virus (HCV) is not recognized as an STD per se. According to the Hepatitis Foundation International, HCV is blood-borne and not easily transmitted sexually. However, people with open lesions from other STDs are at increased risk of acquiring HCV through sexual activity. The Foundation lists multiple sex partners as a risk factor for HCV acquisition and recommends safer sex practices as a safeguard against HCV infection.

HIV/AIDS — You probably already know more about HIV infection and AIDS than we can possibly cover here, but it's nevertheless important to include. HIV is, after all, transmitted primarily through unprotected sexual intercourse, so the precautions required for other STDs can also help to prevent the spread of HIV. As with so many other viral infections, symptoms may not show up until years after the virus takes hold. The symptoms are extremely diverse, mimicking dozens of other illnesses. HIV attacks the immune system itself, wrecking the body's natural defenses against a host of different infections. There are treatments to slow this assault against the immune system, but as yet none suppresses it completely.

While the diseases listed above are the most troublesome STDs in many ways, others are worth mentioning as well.

Common parasites such as *Trichomonas vaginalis,* a frequent cause of vaginitis (inflammation of the vaginal tissue), are often transmitted sexually—to the tune of 5 million new infections annually. There are a dozen other infections easily spread through intimate contact, including sex. These include scabies and lice.

If you want more information about any or all sexually transmitted infections, there are a number of resources to call on. One major source of help is free of charge and as convenient as the nearest telephone: the CDC National STD and AIDS Hotline. (See Resource List, page 221, for this and other useful phone numbers and Web sites.) The CDC hotline offers confidential information and referrals, including print materials sent free of charge to your home address. It also can tell you the location of an STD clinic run by the public health department in your community. Testing and treatment for STDs is often free or inexpensive.

AN OUNCE OF PREVENTION

Because there are so many epidemic STDs, it's critical that you learn to minimize the risk of either getting or spreading these diseases. STDs are transmitted in a variety of ways, but a few principles of prevention apply equally to almost all of them:

> • Most STDs can have mild or unrecognized symptoms. Therefore you can't assume that a lack of symptoms equals a clean bill of health.

> • Testing for the leading STDs is not a routine part of regular healthcare for most people. Don't assume you have been tested for anything. Ask your healthcare

provider about specific tests for chlamydia, gonorrhea, HIV, and herpes. In addition, regular Pap smears are your best line of defense against complications from HPV infection. If a Pap smears show abnormalities, additional HPV testing may be helpful.

• If you're free of infection yourself, your risk is zero if you have sex only with one *uninfected* partner, who in turn has sex only with you. As soon as either partner has a new sexual contact, however, all bets are off. With so many STDs that show no symptoms, how do you know who is infected and who isn't?

• What if you don't really know your partner well and certainly don't know about his or her past? Those having sex with a partner who *might* be carrying an STD, or with several such partners, can dramatically reduce their risk of getting or spreading an STD by using condoms for each and every act of sexual intercourse—whether the penetration is oral, vaginal, or anal. Condoms used in this way are very effective prevention for chlamydia, gonorrhea, syphilis, hepatitis, and HIV. For STDs spread through direct contact with skin lesions, such as herpes and HPV, condoms offer less thorough protection but are still considered useful.

HERPES AND OTHER STDS

Some people with herpes question whether they are at greater risk of getting other illnesses because of HSV. Some assume that a person with one virus in the herpes family will be prone to get all of them. Others have seen press coverage which implies herpes might somehow mutate into the AIDS virus or that herpes itself will damage the immune system or cause cancer.

On all of these points, the facts should be reassuring. Because all the herpesviruses are quite common, you may host herpes simplex and several other members of the family as well, such as Epstein-Barr and varicella zoster. But having HSV in no way dooms you to getting all the herpesviruses; each one is transmitted separately. Nor does having HSV mean that you have a deficient immune system.

Lastly, herpes does not cause cancer, nor does it turn into HIV, although it may make a person more susceptible to contracting HIV. Actually, several of the other STDs mentioned in this chapter are also considered risk factors for HIV. Chlamydia, gonorrhea, syphilis—the presence of any of these infections increases the risk of acquiring HIV, *if and when* there is sexual contact with an HIV-infected person. But none of them by itself leads to HIV. (By the way, it's probable that a person with HIV is more infectious if he or she has another STD as well.)

There is also what some experts call a behavioral linkage between HIV and other sexually transmitted infections. In other words, if you already have an STD, there is a good chance you had unprotected sex with others who have had unprotected sex. Therefore, in statistical terms, anyone with an STD has an increased risk for HIV. It's important to note that the combination of alcohol use and sexual activity may also be considered a risk factor for HIV and other STDs, since alcohol can cloud judgment and lead to unprotected sex. These generalizations may or may not apply to you personally, but they are worth considering seriously. If you have doubts about your HIV status you can learn more about testing by calling the CDC National STD and AIDS Hotline (see Resources, page 223).

WHAT YOU CAN DO

If you have herpes, you now know that sexually transmitted infections are real and present in your life as well as in millions of other lives. Call the CDC National STD and AIDS Hotline (see Resources, page 223) for more information about STDs, for free written materials, or for referral to a healthcare provider in your community. If you feel you may have been exposed to other STDs through unprotected sex, or if you have symptoms that resemble those of a common STD, talk to your healthcare provider about it. There are tests for all the infections listed here. And as always, early treatment is the key to avoiding serious medical complications.

MANAGING HERPES

19

LEGAL ISSUES

❀

"I was dating this girl, and we slept together once," says a caller to the National Herpes Hotline. "Now I've got herpes, and I'm thinking about taking legal action. I'm sure I got it from her. Is there any way I can prove it?"

If you've already read the first 18 chapters of this book, you know that this caller has a lot to learn about herpes, starting with the fact that he probably can't be sure how he became infected at all. This uncertainty is pretty common with regard to other STDs as well.

Lawsuits waged by one person against another over sexually transmitted infections are often pointless. Not only is it difficult (if not impossible) to prove when and from whom the injured party contracted a particular STD, it may be equally difficult to establish that the "guilty" party even knew he or she was infected. What's more, such cases invade the privacy of both plaintiff and defendant and can be a wrenching experience for everyone involved. Nonetheless, questions about herpes and the courts do come up from time to time, and you may want to know a bit about the legal landscape.

COMMON LAW AND INFECTIOUS DISEASES

On the rise since the mid-1980s, lawsuits over sexually transmitted infections generally involve principles of *common law* as opposed to *statutory law*.

Statutory law is usually the product of legislation. Most statutory law is criminal law. The plaintiff is usually the local, state, or federal government, and the penalties include such measures as fines and jail sentences. For example, a number of states have passed laws making it a crime to knowingly pass HIV (the AIDS virus) to another person. In fact, the Ryan White Act of 1990, which provides emergency AIDS grants to states, requires states receiving those funds to make it a crime for HIV-infected people not to tell potential sex partners about their HIV status.

Common law, on the other hand, is generally not legislated but is based on a complex tradition of legal and moral principles as interpreted by the courts over time. The plaintiff in such cases is usually an individual, and the penalties are usually monetary. Thus, if Jimmy wrongs Johnny, Johnny can sue, and it's up to the court to decide if Johnny is entitled to monetary compensation. How do the courts make such determinations? They consider the arguments on both sides and refer to legal precedent within their state. As a result, the rules can vary quite a bit from one state to another.

People have long been held liable in common-law cases for exposing others to infectious diseases such as tuberculosis and whooping cough. In 1896, for example, the Wisconsin Supreme Court ruled that an employer should have told a servant that the employer's child was sick with typhoid fever before the servant cleaned the child's room. And in the 1920 case *Crowell v. Crowell,* the North Carolina Supreme Court held that a man was liable for fraudulently concealing from his bride that he had syphilis. In the modern era, the same type of legal argument has been applied to infectious agents such as HIV, herpes simplex, and human papillomavirus. Because of its deadly consequences, lawsuits involving HIV infection have attracted greater publicity than other STD cases, but there have been some heavily publicized herpes cases as well.

Given the complex patchwork of local and state jurisdictions, no one knows how many STD cases are pending at any given time, but experts say that only a small percentage ever reach the courtroom.

THE LEGAL FRAMEWORK

If and when someone decides to launch a legal action over becoming infected with an STD, he or she generally pursues one of several common strategies. Some have sued for *assault* or *infliction of emotional distress*; others have sued for *fraud, misrepresentation*, or *criminal negligence*. Whatever the line of argument, however, these cases usually hinge on the issue of candor. Did the defendant know he or she had an STD? If not, did he or she take reasonable care to discover this condition? Did he or she withhold this information? And in doing so, did the defendant either accidentally or intentionally harm an innocent person?

While courts in various states might differ on the subtleties of interpretation in STD cases, the growing number of cases settled in recent years is creating a legal consensus that *a person has a legal right to know about the health of a sex partner*. Thus in the eyes of the court, those with an STD have a duty to disclose that fact to those with whom they are sexually intimate. Lying to conceal an STD is often considered a form of *intentional infliction of harm*. Simply failing to tell a partner about an STD, on the other hand, is more likely to be viewed as an act of *negligence*.

By the very nature of the supposed wrongdoing, cases involving the transmission of STDs are difficult to prove. Things were said or not said, actions were taken or not taken—all in the heat of passion and rarely before witnesses.

In terms of physical evidence, the plaintiff often has a tough time establishing causation—proving that the defendant was the cause of the plaintiff's infection. With herpes, as we know, the infection may be acquired months or years before symptoms appear or are recognized. And more than half of all transmission occurs when a partner is asymptomatic or has symptoms but doesn't recognize them as herpes. If the plaintiff has had more than one partner, it may be impossible to prove that an infection came from a particular person. Pinpointing the source is, at the least, very difficult, and medical evidence must be supported by laboratory documentation of a first episode of HSV infection.

COMMON DEFENSES

Tracing the source of several other sexually transmitted infections can be equally challenging, so most defendants in STD cases avail themselves of expert opinion to challenge the proof of the claims made against them. As part of this process, the sexual past of the plaintiff often becomes an issue. Questions raised by the defense attorney will probably include the prior sexual history of the plaintiff and may well overstep our usual notions of privacy and propriety.

In addition, defense lawyers in some of these cases have used strategies to question the very basis of the lawsuit. In some states, for example, it's a criminal offense for people to have sexual relations outside of marriage (defined legally as *fornication*). In these states, the courts have sometimes ruled that a plaintiff cannot recover damages that occurred during an illegal act. Alternately, the defense will sometimes seek protection in laws that offer spousal immunity, making claims between spouses a moot point.

These defense strategies continue to be used in some jurisdictions; however, the trend is to see them both as somewhat antiquated legal notions. In general, the courts have ruled that unmarried persons can sue their sexual partners. California's *Kathleen K. v. Robert B.* set several precedents. The defendant argued that single people do not have a relationship of trust and confidence like married people, but the court ruled that intimate acts imply such a relationship. The defendant also argued that the plaintiff assumed the risk of getting an STD when she had intercourse, but the court said, essentially, that consent to intercourse is *not* consent to being infected with an STD.

This last point is perhaps the most hotly contested in the legal arena. Some defense attorneys have been able to argue persuasively that anyone who has unprotected sexual intercourse in today's society, or who fails to ask about the sexual health of a partner, is equally responsible for infections that may be transmitted sexually, especially during a one-night stand. In less casual relationships, however, the courts are more likely to see a lack of candor as a breach of trust.

Lawyers have found a great many subtleties in STD cases, and the legal landscape is still taking shape. There is, however, growing consensus about the importance of honest disclosure. If someone with an STD tells his or her partner in a meaningful way and gives the partner a choice about sexual involvement, grounds for legal action are vastly reduced. If, on the other hand, someone lies about or conceals the truth about his or her infection, there is ample precedent to suggest he or she might be vulnerable in a legal action.

HERPES AND HEALTH INSURANCE

Slightly more common than questions about lawsuits are concerns about health insurance and the potential for discrimination. Overall, the news here is good. For the nearly two-thirds of Americans covered under a group plan as part of their employee benefits, herpes generally is no issue at all. Millions of people with genital HSV routinely submit claims for office visits, prescription medication, and sometimes counseling. There may be limits placed on coverage under any particular policy, but herpes is seldom, if ever, regarded as different from other medical conditions.

Problems do sometimes emerge, however, for people who seek health insurance for themselves outside large group plans. If you're applying for coverage as part of an individual or family plan, or as part of a small business plan with fewer than 25 participants, you may have to file a detailed application that includes questions about STDs. And for some insurers, a history of herpes or other sexually transmitted infections may prompt further questions.

Some small plans will regard herpes as a *pre-existing condition*, just as they would many other illnesses. In this case, they would enroll you but would exclude herpes-related claims until some waiting period has passed. Others may accept you as a plan member but attach a *rider* to the policy that excludes coverage for herpes altogether. There's also a small chance that your application to a small group may be rejected.

Currently, most insurance companies examine individual or small group applications on a case-by-case basis and make decisions according to a variety of factors. Industry sources say that a history of herpes alone would seldom be grounds for denying coverage. It's also important to remember that herpes claims have almost insignificant cost when compared with diabetes, heart disease, and many other ailments.

Anyone who has questions about health insurance or about discrimination in this area can take one of several steps:

• Work with an experienced, independent insurance agent who knows the insurance companies in your state and can provide a list of companies that accept people with genital herpes.

• Consumers can contact the A.M. Best Company for annually updated ratings of life and health insurers. (Ratings reflect the financial stability of these companies.) A.M. Best can be reached at (908) 439-2200 or at www.ambest.com.

• Some states have *open enrollment programs* in which applicants cannot be denied coverage for medical reasons. Your state department of insurance will have detailed information about these.

• If you have problems getting coverage, you can appeal the insurance company's decision in writing. We know of several cases in which the original decision was overturned solely on the basis of consumer protest. You also have the legal right of access to your MIB (Medical Information Bureau) file, which insurers routinely review as part of their background check on individuals applying for coverage. MIB, Inc. is a nonprofit industry "alliance" whose membership comprises more than 600 health insurance companies. It was originally established to root out fraudulent health insurance claims. MIB keeps files on only a small percentage of insured individuals.

To find out if you have an MIB file and to obtain a copy if you do, contact MIB, Inc. The mailing address is MIB, Inc., P.O. Box 105, Essex Station, Boston, MA 02112. However, *we strongly recommend that you visit the MIB website first*, if possible, at www.mib.com. There you'll find detailed information on the organization and its mission as well as instructions on how to request your records. You can also download the necessary information request form, which will save you a lot of time. As of this writing (March 2001), the fee for record search and disclosure, which can be waived under special circumstances, is $8.50.

RESOURCE LIST

ASHA SERVICES AND MATERIALS

The American Social Health Association (ASHA) has operated the Herpes Resource Center since 1979. To order materials or to find out more about ASHA's services and publications, call the National Herpes Hotline, visit the ASHA Web site (www.ashastd.org), or write:

ASHA/HRC
P.O. Box 13827
Research Triangle Park, NC 27709-3827

NATIONAL HERPES HOTLINE (919-361-8488). The National Herpes Hotline (NHH) operates Monday through Friday, 9 AM to 7 PM Eastern Time. Information specialists are available to address questions related to diagnosis, transmission, prevention, and treatment of herpes simplex virus. The NHH also takes orders for print materials including ASHA's quarterly newsletter on herpes, *the helper*, and provides referrals to a network of local support groups.

THE HELPER. Now in its 23rd year, this quarterly journal covers herpes simplex virus (HSV) topics ranging from symptoms to psychosocial issues to treatment options. Each issue updates readers on leading clinical research and also provides a forum for personal perspectives on HSV. Back issues of *the helper* are also available. Order online or by phone (919-361-8488).

UNDERSTANDING HERPES. A 16-page overview, designed primarily for the newly diagnosed patient, that explains how herpes is transmitted, symptoms, treatment issues, herpes in pregnancy, and how to deal with psychosocial pressures.

ASHA WEB SITE: The ASHA site (www.ashastd.org) offers an in-depth FAQ section, a herpes chat room, an e-mail service to answer specific questions, and access to online ordering for print materials on herpes. Hotline resources and local support group listings are also posted on the site.

HELP GROUPS. The Herpes Resource Center (HRC) coordinates a network of local support groups (called HELP Groups) throughout the United States, Canada, and Australia. These allow participants living with herpes to share experiences, information, and support in an empathetic environment.

HSV RESEARCH. The American Social Health Association (ASHA) Research Fund supports research on HSV and other sexually transmitted diseases. Since 1975, ASHA has sponsored postdoctoral fellows to research biomedical and clinical aspects of HSV, including vaccines.

STD HOTLINES

National STD Hotline (800) 227-8922
(24 hours/day, 7 days/week)

National AIDS Hotline
English Service (800) 342-AIDS
(24 hours/day, 7 days/week)

Spanish Service (800) 344-7432
(8 AM – 2 AM, ET, 7 days/week)

TTY Service for the Deaf (800) 243-7889
(10 AM - 10 PM, ET, M - F)

National HPV & Cervical Cancer Prevention Hotline
(919) 361-4848
(2 PM – 7 PM, ET, M - F)

INFORMATION ON MEDICATIONS

United States Food and Drug Administration (FDA) Office of Consumer Affairs
5600 Fishers Lane
Rockville, MD 20857
1-888-463-6332
www.fda.gov
The FDA provides information on a wide array of topics, including prescription medications, over-the-counter drugs,

dietary supplements, vaccines, and medical devices (including condoms). Of particular note is the Drug Information Hotline of the FDA Center for Drug Evaluation and Research: (301) 827-4573.

GlaxoSmithKline

5 Moore Drive
Research Triangle Park, NC 27709
(888) 825-5249
www.herpeshelp.com
As the maker of the antiviral medication Valtrex®, GlaxoSmithSkline maintains both a Web site and a consumer hotline that can direct callers to information specialists and to company programs such as the Patient Assistance Program.

Novartis Pharmaceuticals

One Health Plaza
East Hanover, NJ 07936-1080
(866) 326-8471
www.healthandhope.com
www.famvir.com
Consumer information about the antiviral medication Famvir® is available from Novartis Pharmaceuticals through the Web sites and hotline listed above.

OTHER RESOURCES

For diagnostic tests:
Diagnology
(877) 229-5210
www.pockit.com

Focus Technologies
800-445-4032
www.focusanswers.com

University of Washington
(206) 598-6066 (healthcare providers only)
http://depts.washington.edu/herpes/

For support and counseling:
American Association of Marriage and Family Therapists
1100 17th St., NW , 10th Floor
Washington, DC 20036
(202) 452-0109, 9 AM – 5 PM, ET, M - F
www.aamft.org
The Association provides information through the mail about therapists in your area. Referrals are for solution-oriented therapy/counseling.

For nutrition information:
American Dietetic Association
(800) 366-1655
www.eatright.org
The ADA's Nutrition Information Line offers referrals to registered dieticians in your area as well as recorded messages

dealing with topics such as exercise and its effect on weight loss. These are varied monthly.

For reproductive health/family planning questions:
Planned Parenthood Federation of America
(800) 829-7732
www.plannedparenthood.org
The Planned Parenthood toll-free number automatically refers callers to the nearest affiliated clinic. Local chapters may provide information over the phone and free pamphlets for men and women.

For information about insurance companies:
A.M. Best Co.
(908) 439-2200
www.ambest.com
This organization provides financial stability ratings of approximately 1,500 insurers.

For information about alternative treatments:
The National Center for Complementary and Alternative Medicine (NCCAM)
National Institutes of Health
(888) 644-6226
http://nccam.nih.gov/
NCCAM explores complementary and alternative healing practices in the context of rigorous science and disseminates authoritative information. Its clearinghouse produces fact

sheets, a newsletter, and other publications that provide information about research supported by the NCCAM and other centers of the NIH. The information is free of charge and can be ordered through the toll-free number listed above.

HERPES-RELATED WEB SITES

There are dozens of Web sites offering resources for people with genital herpes, but Web surfers cannot always count on the quality of the information presented. The sites listed here are among the most thorough, with an emphasis on content grounded in published scientific research. For a much more complete listing of sites, check the Links page on the ASHA Web site listed below.

American Social Health Association (ASHA)

www.ashastd.org

The ASHA site offers an in-depth FAQ section, a herpes chat room, an e-mail service to answer specific questions, and access to online ordering for print materials on herpes. Hotline resources and local support group listings are also posted on the site.

American Herpes Foundation

www.herpes-foundation.org

Information and resources for patients and medical professionals.

HerpesWeb

www.herpesweb.net

Well-designed international site with patient resources, personal accounts.

International Herpes Alliance

www.herpesalliance.com

Educational pages, news, resources, and personal accounts from patients around the world.

International Herpes Management Forum

www.ihmf.org

International academic organization that addresses the clinical care of all major herpesvirus infections. Includes HSV information for patient and professional.

National Institutes of Health (NIH)

www.niaid.nih.gov/factsheets/stdherp.htm

or www.nih.gov

The consumer–oriented "Healthfinder" service available through the NIH Web site offers a question-and-answer page geared to those diagnosed with genital herpes.

U.S. Centers for Disease Control and Prevention (CDC)

www.cdc.gov

or www.cdc.gov/nchstp/dstd/Fact_Sheets/facts_Genital_Herpes.htm

CDC's Sexually Transmitted Diseases Branch publishes a herpes fact sheet online, along with a bibliography of references and a listing of resources.

WebMD Genital Herpes Chat
http://my.webmd.com/roundtable_topic/90
Bulletin board of postings and chat, with questions answered by herpes expert Terri Warren, R.N., A.N.P., M.S.

GLOSSARY

ACUTE OR EPISODIC THERAPY: Use of medication to relieve symptoms or hasten healing for an individual herpes outbreak.

ANTIBODIES: Elements of the body's immune response, antibodies circulate in the blood and in other bodily fluids to fight disease-causing microbes.

ANTIGEN: Any foreign substance in the body, such as a fragment of a virus, that triggers the immune system to respond with antibodies or other parts of the immune defense system.

ASYMPTOMATIC REACTIVATION, ASYMPTOMATIC SHEDDING: An event in which latent herpes simplex virus reactivates at the nerve root and travels to a skin surface or mucous membrane, yet causes neither signs nor symptoms of infection that can be readily identified by the patient or a medical professional.

ASYMPTOMATIC TRANSMISSION: The spread of virus from one person to another during a period of asymptomatic shedding.

AUTOINOCULATION: The spread of HSV from one part of the body to another. This can result when a person with active herpes deposits a significant amount of virus onto some other vulnerable part of the body—most often a mucous membrane.

CELL CULTURE (VIRAL CULTURE): A diagnostic test for many kinds of viruses. In a cell culture for HSV, a swab of the patient's herpes lesion is placed in a laboratory dish containing normal skin cells to see if HSV will grow.

CELLULAR IMMUNE RESPONSE: The portion of the body's immune response that involves T-lymphocytes—specialized or other cells designed to fight an "antigen" or invading microbe.

DISSEMINATED INFECTION: A herpes infection that spreads over a wider than usual area of the body, frequently afflicting internal organs.

FIRST EPISODE: The body's first encounter with a particular type of herpes simplex, an event that often produces marked symptoms. There are two types of "first episodes." A primary first episode describes the symptoms that appear in the person who has never been infected with either HSV-1 or HSV-2 before. It's sometimes called a "true primary," and it tends to be most severe.

"Nonprimary first episode" describes the symptoms that occur in the person who has been infected first with one type of HSV and then later infected with the second. For example, a person who is infected with HSV-1 and then years later infected with HSV-2 can be said to have a "first episode" of HSV-2 if he or she has symptoms.

"First recognized recurrence" describes the first episode of genital herpes in a person who has had the infection for some time but has not noticed the symptoms in the past.

GANGLION: A knot-like grouping of the nerves that serve a particular part of the body.

GENITAL HERPES: "Genital herpes" can cause symptoms in a variety of sites below the waist. This term is used to denote all HSV infection that is latent in the sacral ganglion, at the base of the spine.

HSV: Abbreviation for herpes simplex virus. HSV-1 denotes herpes simplex type 1, the usual cause of herpes around the mouth or face ("cold sores," "fever blisters"); HSV-2 denotes herpes simplex type 2, the usual cause of recurrent genital herpes.

HERPES ENCEPHALITIS: A rare severe illness that occurs when the brain becomes infected with HSV.

HERPES GLADIATORUM: The presence of herpes lesions on the body skin caused by HSV infection that is transmitted usually through the abrasion of skin in a contact sport, such as wrestling.

HERPES WHITLOW: The presence of herpes lesions on the fingers or toes near the nailbed.

HERPESVIRUS: Any one of eight known members of the human herpesvirus family: herpes simplex type 1; herpes simplex type 2; varicella zoster virus; Epstein-Barr virus; cytomegalovirus; human herpes virus type 6; human herpes virus type 7; and human herpes virus type 8.

LATENCY: The phenomenon by which HSV can persist in the nerve roots in an inactive state but retain the capacity to reactivate intermittently and cause viral shedding and lesions.

LESION: A very general term denoting any abnormality on the surface of the body, whether on the skin or on a mucous membrane. Includes sores, pimples, tumors, and more.

MENINGITIS: An inflammation of the meninges, the protective covering around the brain, usually accompanied by stiff neck and extra sensitivity to light. Septic meningitis, caused by bacteria, can be a serious condition and must be treated immediately. Aseptic meningitis, associated with viral infections such as HSV and other causes, generally resolves by itself.

OCULAR HERPES: Symptoms caused by herpes infection in the eyes.

ORAL-FACIAL HERPES: The presence of latent herpes simplex infection in the trigeminal ganglion, at the top of the spine.

When reactivated, oral-facial herpes can cause symptoms anywhere on mouth or face—typically cold sores on the lips. Recurrent oral-facial herpes is caused almost exclusively by HSV-1.

PRODROME: An early warning symptom of illness, prodrome for a genital herpes outbreak often involves an aching, burning, itching, or tingling sensation in the genital area, buttocks, or legs.

PRODRUG: A medication that must undergo chemical conversion in the body in order to change to its active form.

RECURRENCE: The presence of lesions caused by reactivation of HSV ("outbreak").

STD: Sexually transmitted disease; any infection that is acquired through sexual contact in a substantial number of cases.

SACRAL GANGLION: The nerve root at the base of the spine that serves as the site of latency in genital herpes infections.

SEROLOGIC TEST: A test that identifies the antibodies in serum (a clear fluid that is a component of blood).

SEROSTATUS: A determination, based on serology, of whether a person has antibodies to any particular microbe—for example, HSV-1 or HSV-2.

STEROIDS: A group of drugs, including corticosteroids and ana-
bolic steroids, that affect metabolism.

SYMPTOMATIC REACTIVATION: The presence of lesions or any
other symptoms caused by reactivation of HSV; a "recurrence."

SYSTEMIC SYMPTOMS: Fever, headache, fatigue, or other symptoms of illness affecting the whole body, as distinguished
from the surface lesions seen in a herpes recurrence.

TRANSMISSION: The spread of herpes from one person to another.

TRIGGER (FACTOR): Any biologic or behavioral event that
influences latent HSV to reactivate.

TRUE PRIMARY EPISODE: A person's first infection with either
type of HSV: a primary first episode. See "first episode."

VIRAL REPLICATION: The process by which a virus makes more
copies of itself.

FURTHER READING

OVERVIEW OF GENITAL HERPES

Benedetti, J., Corey, L., Ashley, R. "Recurrence Rates in Genital Herpes after Symptomatic First-Episode Infections." *Annals of Internal Medicine* 1994; 12: 847-54.

Benedetti, J.K., Zeh, J., Corey, L., "Clinical reactivation of genital herpes simplex virus infection decreases in frequency over time." *Annals of Internal Medicine* 1999; 131(1): 14-20.

Benedetti, J., Zeh, J., Selke, S., Corey, L. "Frequency and Reactivation of Nongenital Lesions among Patients with Genital Herpes Simplex Virus." *American Journal of Medicine* 1995; 98: 237.

Brock, V.B., Selke, S., Benedetti, J., Douglas, J., Corey, L. "Frequency of Asymptomatic Shedding of Herpes Simplex Virus in Women with Genital Herpes." *JAMA* 1990; 263: 418-20.

Centers for Disease Control and Prevention, Division of STD Prevention. "Sexually Transmitted Disease Surveillance 1995." Atlanta: U.S. Department of Health and Human Services, Public Health Service, Sept. 1996.

Corey, L. "The Current Trend in Genital Herpes: Progress in Prevention." *Sexually Transmitted Diseases* (Supplement 2) Mar/Apr 1994; 21: S38-S44.

Corey, L. "Genital Herpes." *Sexually Transmitted Diseases.* Second Edition. Ed. K. Holmes. New York: McGraw-Hill, 1990: 392-6.

Corey, L., Adams, H., Brown, Z., Holmes, K. "Genital Herpes Virus Simplex Infections: Clinical Manifestations, Course, and Complications." *Annals of Internal Medicine* 1983; 98: 958-72.

Corey, L., Handsfield, H., "Genital Herpes and Public Health." *JAMA* 2000; 283(6): 791-794.

Corey, L., Spear, P. "Infections with Herpes Simplex Viruses (1)." *New England Journal of Medicine* 1986; 314(11): 686-91.

Corey, L., Spear, P. "Infections with Herpes Simplex Viruses (2)." *New England Journal of Medicine* 1986; 314(12): 749-57.

Fleming, D., McQuillan, G., Johnson, R., Nahmias, A., Aral, S., Lee, F., St. Louis, M. "Herpes Simplex Virus Type 2 in the United States, 1976 to 1994." *New England Journal of Medicine* 1997; 337(16): 1105-11.

Lafferty, W., Coombs, R., Benedetti, J., Critchlow, C., Corey, L. "Recurrences after Oral and Genital Herpes Simplex Virus Infection: Influence of Site of Infection and Viral Type." *New England Journal of Medicine* 1987; 316(23): 1444-9.

Langenberg, A., Benedetti, J., Jenkins, J., Ashley, R., Winter, C., Corey, L. "Development of Clinically Recognizable Lesions among Women Previously Identified as Having 'Asymptomatic' Herpes Simplex Virus Type 2 Infection." *Annals of Internal Medicine* 1989; 110(11): 882-7.

Langenberg, A., Corey, L., Ashley, R., Leong, W.P., Straus, S., "A Prospective Study of New Infections with Herpes Simplex Virus Type 1 and Type 2." *New England Journal of Medicine* 1999; 341: 19: 1432-1438.

Koelle, D., Benedetti, J., Langenberg, A., Corey, L. "Asymptomatic Reactivation of Herpes Simplex Virus in Women after the First Episode of Genital Herpes." *Annals of Internal Medicine* 1992; 116: 433-7.

Kost, R., Straus, S. "Postherpetic Neuralgia: Pathogenesis, Treatment, and Prevention." *New England Journal of Medicine* 1996; 335(1): 32-42.

Mertz, G. "Epidemiology of Genital Herpes Infections." *Infectious Disease Clinics of North America* 1993; 7: 825-39.

Mertz, G. "Genital Herpes Simplex Virus Infections." *Medical Clinics of North America* 1990; 74(6): 1433-51.

Nahmias, A., Lee, F., Beckman-Nahmias, S. "Seroepidemiological and Sociological Patterns of Herpes Simplex Virus Infection in the World." *Scandinavian Journal of Infectious Diseases* (Supplement) 1990; 69: 19-36.

Reeves, W., Corey, L., Adams, H., Vontver, L., Holmes, K. "Risk of Recurrence after First Episodes of Genital Herpes: Relation to HSV Type and Antibody Response." *New England Journal of Medicine* 1981; 305(6): 315-9.

Sacks, S. *The Truth About Herpes.* Fourth Edition. Seattle: Gordon Soules, 1997.

Sacks, S. "Frequency and Duration of Patient-Observed Recurrent Genital Herpes Simplex Virus Infection: Characterization of the Nonlesional Prodrome." *Journal of Infectious Diseases* 1984; 150: 873-7.

Wald, A., Corey, L., Cone, R., Hobson, A., Davis, G., Zeh, J. "Frequent Genital Herpes Simplex Virus 2 Shedding in Immunocompetent Women: Effect of Acyclovir Treatment." *Journal of Clinical Investigation* 1997; 99(5): 1092-7.

Wald, A., Zeh, J., Selke, S., "Reactivation of genital herpes simplex virus type 2 infection in asymptomatic HSV-2 seropositive persons." *New England Journal of Medicine* 2000; 342: 844-850.

Wald, A., Zeh, J., Selke, S., Ashley, R., Corey, L. "Virologic Characteristics of Subclinical and Symptomatic Genital Herpes Infection." *New England Journal of Medicine* 1995; 333: 770-5.

Whitley, R., Gnann, J. "The Epidemiology and Clinical Manifestations of Herpes Simplex Virus Infections." *The Human Herpesviruses.* Ed. B. Roizman, R. Whitley, and C. Lopez. New York: Raven Press, 1993.

THE FAMILY OF HERPESVIRUSES

Berneman, Z., Ablashi, L., Eger-Fletcher, M., Reitz, M., Hung, C., Brus, I., Komaroff, A., Gallo, R. "Human Herpesvirus 7 Is a T-Lymphotropic Virus and Relates to, but Is Significantly Different from, Human Herpesvirus 6 and Human Cytomegalovirus." *Proceedings of the National Academy of Sciences* 1992; 89: 10552.

Levy, J. "Three New Human Herpesviruses (HHV6, 7, and 8)." *Lancet* 1997; 349(9051): 558-63.

Roizman, B. "The Family Herpesviridae: A Brief Introduction." *The Human Herpesviruses.* Ed. B. Roizman, R. Whitley, and C. Lopez. New York: Raven Press, 1993.

Spear, P. "Biology of the Herpesviruses." *Sexually Transmitted Diseases.* Second Edition. Ed. K. Holmes. New York: McGraw-Hill, 1990: 379-80.

Weller, T. "Varicella and Herpes Zoster: Changing Concepts of the Natural History, Control, and Importance of a Not-So-Benign Virus." *New England Journal of Medicine* 1983; 309(22): 1362-8.

Wolk, S. "The Nature and Diagnosis of Clinically Important Viruses." *Physician Assistant* Jun 1993: 23-24.

TRANSMISSION AND PREVENTION

Abesfeld, D., Thomas, I. "Cutaneous Herpes Simplex Virus Infection." *American Family Practice* 1991; 43(5): 1655.

Bryson, Y., Dillon, M., Bernstein, D., Radolf, J., Zakowski, P., Garratty, E. "Risk of Acquisition of Genital Herpes Simplex Virus Type 2 in Sex Partners of Persons with Genital Herpes: A Prospective Couple Study." *Journal of Infectious Diseases* 1993; 167: 942-6.

Centers for Disease Control and Prevention. "Update: Barrier Protection Against HIV Infection and Other Sexually Transmitted Diseases." *MMWR* 1993; 42(30).

Corey, L., Langenberg, A. G., Ashley, R., et al. "Recombinant glycoprotein vaccine for the prevention of genital HSV-2 infection: two randomized controlled trials." *JAMA* 1999; 282(4): 331-40.

Douglas, J., Corey, L. "Fomites and Herpes Simplex Viruses: A Case for Nonvenereal Transmission?" *JAMA* 1983; 250(22): 3093-4.

Judson, F., Ehret, J., Bodin, G., Levin, M., Reitmeijer, C. "In Vitro Evaluation of Condoms with and without Nonoxynol 9 as Physical and Chemical Barriers Against Chlamydia trachomatis, Herpes Simplex Virus Type 2, and Human Immunodeficiency Virus." *Sexually Transmitted Diseases* 1989; 16(2): 51-54.

Koutsky, L., Ashley, R., Holmes, K., Stevens, C., Critchlow, C., Kiviat, N., Lipinski, C., Wolner-Hanssen, P., Corey, L. "The Frequency of Unrecognized Type 2 Herpes Simplex Virus Infections among Women:

Implications for Control of Genital Herpes." *Sexually Transmitted Diseases* Apr/Jun 1990; 17(2): 90-94.

Mertz, G., Benedetti, J., Ashley, R., Selke, S., Corey, L. "Risk Factors for the Sexual Transmission of Genital Herpes." *Annals of Internal Medicine* 1992; 116: 197-202.

Mertz, G., Coombs, R., Ashley, R., Jourden, J., Remington, M., Winter, C., Fahnlander, A., Guinan, M., Ducey, H., and Corey, L. "Transmission of Genital Herpes in Couples with One Symptomatic and One Asymptomatic Partner: A Prospective Study." *Journal of Infectious Diseases* 1988; 157(6): 1169-77.

Mertz, G., Schmidt, O., Jourden, J., Guinan, M., Remington, M., Fahnlander, A., Winter, C., Holmes, K., Corey, L. "Frequency of Acquisition of First-Episode Genital Infection with Herpes Simplex Virus from Symptomatic and Asymptomatic Source Contacts." *Sexually Transmitted Diseases* Jan/Mar 1985; 12(1): 33-39.

Rooney, J., Felser, J., Ostrove, J., Straus, S. "Acquisition of Genital Herpes from an Asymptomatic Sexual Partner." *New England Journal of Medicine* 1986; 314(24): 1563.

Wald, A., Zeh, J., Barnum, G., Davis, G., Corey, L. "Suppression of Subclinical Shedding of Herpes Simplex Virus Type 2 with Acyclovir." *Annals of Internal Medicine* 1996; 124: 8-15.

TREATMENT OPTIONS

Bryson, Y., Dillon, M., Lovett, M., Acuna, G., Taylor, S., Cherry, J., Johnson, L., Wiesmeier, E., Growdon, W., Creagh-Kirk, T., Keeney, R. "Treatment of First Episodes of Genital Herpes Simplex Virus Infection with Oral Acyclovir: A Randomized Double-Blind Controlled Trial in Normal Subjects." *New England Journal of Medicine* Apr 1983; 308: 916-21.

Centers for Disease Control and Prevention. "Sexually Transmitted Diseases Treatment Guidelines." *MMWR* 1998; 47 (No. RR-1).

Corey, L., Nahmias, A., Guinan, M., Benedetti, J., Critchlow, C., Holmes, K. "A Trial of Topical Acyclovir in Genital Herpes Simplex Virus Infections." *New England Journal of Medicine* 1982; 306: 1313-9.

Dorsky, D., Crumpacker, C. "Drugs Five Years Later: Acyclovir." *Annals of Internal Medicine* 1987; 107: 859-74.

Fife, K., Barbarash, R., Rudolph, T., "Valaciclovir versus acyclovir in the treatment of first-episode genital herpes infection: results of an international, multicenter, double-blind randomized clinical trial." *Sexually Transmitted Diseases* 1997; 24: 481-486.

Fife, K., Crumpacker, C., Mertz, G., Hill, E., Boone, G., and the Acyclovir Study Group. "Recurrence and Resistance Patterns of Herpes Simplex Virus Following Cessation of Greater than or Equal to Six Years of Chronic Suppression with Acyclovir." *Journal of Infectious Diseases* 1994; 169: 1338-41.

Goldberg, L., Kaufman, R., Conant, M., Sperber, J., Allen, M., Illeman, M., Donohew, P., Chapman, S. "Episodic Twice-Daily Treatment for Recurrent Genital Herpes." *American Journal of Medicine* (Supplement 2A) 1988; 85: 10-13.

Goldberg, L., Kaufman, R., Kurtz, T., Conant, M., Eron, L., Batenhorst, R., Boone, G. and the Acyclovir Study Group. "Long-Term Suppression of Recurrent Genital Herpes with Acyclovir: A 5-Year Benchmark." *Archives of Dermatology* 1993; 129: 582-7.

Jacobson, M., Gallant, J., Wang, L., Coakley, D., Weller, S., Gary, D., Squires, L., Smiley, L., Blum, M., Feinberg, J. "Phase I Trial of Valaciclovir, the L-Valyl Ester of Acyclovir, in Patients with Advanced Human

Immunodeficiency Virus Disease." *Antimicrobial Agents and Chemotherapy* 1994; 38(7): 1534-40.

Kaplowitz, L., Baker, D., Gelb, L., Blythe, J., Hale, R., Frost, P., Crumpacker, C., Rabinovich, S., Peacock, J., Herndon, J., Davis, G., and the Acyclovir Study Group. "Prolonged Continuous Acyclovir Treatment of Normal Adults with Frequently Recurring Genital Herpes Simplex Virus Infection." *JAMA* 1991; 256(6): 747-51.

Kost, R., Hill, E., Tigges, M., Straus, S. "Brief Report: Recurrent Acyclovir-Resistant Genital Herpes in an Immunocompetent Patient." *New England Journal of Medicine* 1993; 329(24): 1777-82.

Mertz, G. "Prolonged Continuous Versus Intermittent Oral Acyclovir Treatment in Normal Adults with Frequently Recurring Genital Herpes Simplex Virus Infection." *American Journal of Medicine* (Supplement 2A) 1988; 85: 16.

Mertz, G., Critchlow, C., Benedetti, J., Reichman, R., Dolin, R., Connor, J., Redfield, D., Savoia, M., Richman, D., Tyrrell, D., Miedzinski, L., Portnoy, J., Keeney, R., Corey, L. "Double-Blind Placebo-Controlled Trial of Oral Acyclovir in First-Episode Genital Herpes Simplex Virus Infection." *JAMA* 1984; 252(9): 1147-51.

Mertz, G., Jones, C., Mills, J., Fofe, K., Lemon, S., Stapleton, J., Hill, E., Davis, L., and the Acyclovir Study Group. "Long-Term Acyclovir Suppression of Frequently Recurring Genital Herpes Simplex Virus Infection. A Multicenter Double-Blind Trial." *JAMA* 1988; 260(2): 201-6.

Mertz, G., Loveless, M., Levin, M., Kraus, S., Fowler, S., Goade, D., Tyring, S. "Oral Famciclovir for Suppression of Recurrent Genital Herpes Simplex Virus Infection in Women." *Archives of Internal Medicine* 1997; 157: 343.

Mindel, A., Carney, O., Freris, M., Faherty, A., Patou, G., Williams, P. "Dosage and Safety of Long-Term Suppressive Acyclovir Therapy for Recurrent Genital Herpes." *Lancet* 1988; 1(8591): 926-8.

Nahata, M. "Clinical Use of Antiviral Drugs." *Drug Intelligence and Clinical Pharmacy* 1987; 21(5): 399-405.

Nilsen, A., Aasen, T., Halsos, A., Kinge, B., Tjotta, E., Wikstrom, K., Fiddian, A. "Efficacy of Oral Acyclovir in the Treatment of Initial and Recurrent Genital Herpes." *Lancet* 1982; 2: 571-3.

Patel, R., Bodsworth, N., Wooley, P., Peters, B., Vejlsgaard, G., Saari, S., Gibb, A., Robinson, J., and the International Valaciclovir HSV Study Group. "Valaciclovir for the Suppression of Recurrent HSV Infection: A Placebo-Controlled Study of Once Daily Therapy." *Genitourinary Medicine* 1997; 73: 105-9.

Patel, R., Tyring, S., Strand, A., Price M.J., Grant, D.M., Impact of suppressive antiviral therapy on the health-related quality of life of patients with recurrent genital herpes infection. *Sexually Transmitted Infections* 1999; 75: 398-402.

Reichman, R., Badger, G., Guinan, M., Nahmias, A., Keeney, R., Davis, L., Ashikaga,T., Dolin, R. "Topically Administered Acyclovir in the Treatment of Recurrent Herpes Simplex Genitalis: A Controlled Trial." *Journal of Infectious Diseases* 1983; 147(2): 336-40.

Reichman, R., Badger, G., Mertz, G., Corey, L., Richman, D., Connor, J., Redfield, D., Savoia, M., Oxman, M., Bryson, Y., Tyrrell, D., Portnoy, J., Creigh-Kirk, T., Keeney, R., Ashikaga, T., Dolin, R. "Treatment of Recurrent Genital Herpes Simplex Infections with Oral Acyclovir: In a Controlled Trial." *JAMA* 1984; 251: 2103-7.

Sacks, S., Aoki, F., Diaz-Mitoma, F., Sellors, J., Shafran, S. "Patient-Initiated, Twice-Daily Oral Famciclovir for Early Recurrent Genital Herpes: A Randomized, Double-Blind Multicenter Trial." *JAMA* 1996; 276(1): 44-49.

Safrin, S. "Treatment of Acyclovir Resistant Herpes Simplex Virus in Infections in Patients with AIDS." *Journal of AIDS* (Supplement 1); 1992: S29-32.

Safrin, S., Crumpacker, C., Chatis, P., Davis, R., Hafner, R., Rush, J., Kessler, H., Landry, B., Mills, J., and other members of the AIDS Clinical Trials Group. "A Controlled Trial Comparing Foscarnet with Vidarabine for Acyclovir-Resistant Mucocutaneous Herpes Simplex in the Acquired Immunodeficiency Syndrome." *New England Journal of Medicine* 1991; 325(8): 551-5.

Sollie, E. *Straight Talk With Your Gynecologist: How to Get Answers That Will Save Your Life.* Hillsboro, OR: Beyond Words, 1992.

Spruance, S., Tyring, S., DeGregorio, B., Miller, C., Beutner, K., and the Valaciclovir HSV Study Group. "A Large Scale Placebo-Controlled, Dose-Ranging Trial of Peroral Valaciclovir for Episodic Treatment of Recurrent Herpes Genitalis." *Archives of Internal Medicine* 1996; 156: 1729-35.

Straus, S., Mindell, S., Takiff, H., Rooney, J., Felser, J., Smith, H., Roane, P., Johnson, F., Hallahan, C., Ostrove, J., Nusinoff-Lehrman, S. "Effect of Oral Acyclovir on Symptomatic and Asymptomatic Virus Shedding in Recurrent Genital Herpes." *Sexually Transmitted Diseases* Apr/Jun 1989; 16(2): 107-13.

Wachsman, M. "Focus on Famciclovir: Review of Its Use in Genital Herpes Simplex Virus Therapy." *Formulary* 1995; 30: 587.

Wald, A., Zeh, J., Barnum, G., Davis, G. "Suppression of Subclinical Shedding of Herpes Simplex Virus Type 2 with Acyclovir." *Annals of Internal Medicine* 1996; 124: 8-15.

Whitley, R., Gnann, J. "Acyclovir: A Decade Later." *New England Journal of Medicine* 1992; 327: 782-9.

Whitley, R., Middlebrooks, M., Gnann, J. "Acyclovir: The Past Ten Years." *Advances in Experimental Medicine and Biology* 1990; 278: 243-53.

TAKING CONTROL—THE EMOTIONAL ISSUES

Aral, S., VanderPlate, C., Magder, L. "Recurrent Genital Herpes: What Helps Adjustment?" *Sexually Transmitted Diseases* 1988; 15(3): 164-6.

Brookes, J., Haywood, S., and Green, J. "Adjustment to the psychological and social sequelae of recurrent genital herpes simplex infection." *Genitourinary Medicine* 1993; 69: 384-7.

Carney, O., et al., "A prospective study of the psychological impact on patients with a first episode of genital herpes." *Genitourinary Medicine* 1994; 70: 40-45.

Catotti, D., Clarke, P., Catoe, K. "Herpes Revisited: Still a Cause of Concern." *Sexually Transmitted Diseases* 1993; 20(2): 77-80.

Greenwood, V., Bernstein, R. "Coping with Herpes: The Emotional Problems." Washington, D.C.: The Washington Center for Cognitive-Behavioral Therapy, 1982.

Mindel, A., "Psychological and psychosexual implications of herpes simplex virus infections." *Scand J Infect Dis Suppl* 1996; 100: 27-32.

Swanson, J., Dibble, S., Chenitz, W. "Clinical features and psychosocial factors in young adults with genital herpes." *J Nursing Scholarship* 1995; 27: 16-22.

VanderPlate, C., Aral, S. "Psychosocial Aspects of Genital Herpes Virus Infection." *Health Psychology* 1987; 6(1): 52-72.

WELLNESS AND ALTERNATIVE THERAPIES

Eisenberg, D., Kessler, R., Foster, C., Norlock, F., Calkins, D., Delbanco, T. "Unconventional Medicine in the United States: Prevalence, Costs, and Patterns of Use." *New England Journal of Medicine* 1993; 328(4): 246.

Griffith, R. "Success of L-Lysine Therapy in Frequently Recurrent Herpes Simplex Infection." *Dermatological* 1987; 175: 183-90.

Longo, D. "Psychosocial Treatment for Recurrent Genital Herpes." *Journal of Consulting and Clinical Psychology* 1988; 56(1): 61-66.

Rooney, J., Bryson, Y., Mannix, M., Dillon, M., Wohlenberg, C., Banks, S., Wallington, C., Notkins, A., Straus, S. "Prevention of Ultraviolet-Light-Induced Herpes Labialis by Sunscreen." *Lancet* 1991; 338(8180): 1419-22.

HERPES AND PREGNANCY

Andrews, E., Yankaskas, B., Cordero, J., Schoeffler, K., Hampp, S., and the Acyclovir in Pregnancy Registry Advisory Committee. "Acyclovir in Pregnancy Registry: Six Years' Experience." *Obstetrics and Gynecology* 1992; 79(1): 8.

Arvin, A., Hensleigh, P., Prober, C., Au, D., Yasukawa, L., Wittek, A., Palumbo, P., Paryani, S., Yeager, S. "Failure of Antepartum Maternal Cultures to Predict the Infant's Risk of Exposure to Herpes Simplex Virus at Delivery." *New England Journal of Medicine* 1986; 315(13): 796-800.

Baker, D. "Herpes and Pregnancy: New Management." *Clinical Obstetrics and Gynecology* 1990; 33(2): 253-7.

Binkin, N., Koplan, J. "The High Cost and Low Efficacy of Weekly Viral Cultures for Pregnant Women with Recurrent Genital Herpes: A Reappraisal." *Medical Decision Making* 1989; 9(4): 226-30.

Brown, Z., Benedetti, J., Ashley, R., Burchett, S., Selke, S., Berry, S., Vontver, L., Corey, L. "Neonatal Herpes Simplex Virus Infection in Relation to Asymptomatic Maternal Infection at the Time of Labor." *New England Journal of Medicine* 1991; 324(18): 1249-50.

Brown, Z., Selke, M., Zeh, J., Kopelman, J., Maslow, A., Ashley, R., Watts, H., Berry, S., Herd, M., Corey, L. "The Acquisition of Herpes Simplex Virus during Pregnancy." *New England Journal of Medicine* 1997; 337(8): 509-15.

Brown, Z., Vontver, L., Benedetti, J., Critchlow, C., Hickok, D., Sells, C., Berry, S., Corey, L. "Recurrent Genital Herpes in Pregnancy: Variation of Recurrence Rates by Trimester and Risk Factors Associated with Asymptomatic Viral Shedding." *American Journal of Obstetrics and Gynecology* 1985; 153: 24-30.

Cone, R., Hobson, A., Brown, Z., Ashley, R., Berry, S., Winter, C., Corey, L. "Frequent Detection of Genital Herpes Simplex Virus DNA by Polymerase Chain Reaction among Pregnant Women." *JAMA* 1994; 272: 792-6.

Hardy, K., Arvin, A., Yasukawa, L., Bronzan, R., Lewinsohn, D., Hensleigh, P., Prober, C. "Use of Polymerase Chain Reaction for Successful Identification of Asymptomatic Genital Infection with Herpes Simplex Virus in Pregnant Women at Delivery." *Journal of Infectious Diseases* 1990; 162: 1031-5.

Harger, J., Amortegui, A., Meyer, M., Pazin, G. "Characteristics of Recurrent Genital Herpes Simplex Infections in Pregnant Women." *Obstetrics and Gynecology* 1989; 73(3): 367-72.

Kulhanjian, J., Soroush, V., Au, D., Bronzan, R., Yasukawa, L., Weylman, L., Arvin, A., Prober, C. "Identification of Women at Unsuspected Risk of Primary Infection with Herpes Simplex Virus Type 2 during Pregnancy." *New England Journal of Medicine* 1992; 326(14): 916-20.

Randolph, A., Washington, E., Prober, C. "Cesarean Delivery for Women Presenting with Genital Herpes Lesions: Efficacy, Risks, and Costs. *JAMA* 1993; 270(1): 77.

Scott, L., Sanchez, P., Jackson, G., Zeray, F., Wendel, G. "Acyclovir Suppression to Prevent Cesarean Delivery after First-Episode Genital Herpes." *Obstetrics and Gynecology* 1996; 87(1): 69-73.

Stone, K., Brooks, C., Guinan, M., Alexander, E. "National Surveillance for Neonatal Herpes Simplex Virus Infections." *Sexually Transmitted Diseases* 1989; 16(3): 152.

Suarez, M., Briones, H., Saaevdra, T. "Buttock Herpes: High Risk in Pregnancy." *Journal of Reproductive Medicine* 1991; 36(5): 367-8.

Whitley, R., Arvin, A., Prober, C., Corey, L., Burchett, S., Plotkin, S., Staff, S., Jacobs, R., Powell, D., Nahmias, A., Sumaya, C., Edwards, K., Alford, C., Caddell, G., Soong, S., and the National Institute of Allergy and Infectious Diseases Collaborative Antiviral Study Group. "Predictors of Morbidity and Mortality in Neonates with Herpes Simplex Virus Infections." *New England Journal of Medicine* 1991; 324(7): 450-4.

THE BROADER SPECTRUM OF HSV INFECTION

Arvin, A., Prober, C. "Herpes Simplex Virus Infections." *Pediatrics in Review* 1992; 13(3): 110-1.

Belongia, E., Goodman, J., Holland, E., Andres, C., Homann, S., Mahanti, R., Mizener, M., Erice, A., Osterhold, M. "An Outbreak of Herpes Gladiatorum at a High-School Wrestling Camp." *New England Journal of Medicine* 1991; 325(13): 906-10.

Bergstrom, T., Vahlne, A., Alestig, K., Jeansson, S., Forsgren, M., Lycke, E. "Primary and Recurrent Herpes Simplex Virus Type 2-Induced Meningitis." *Journal of Infectious Diseases* 1990; 162: 327.

Deschenes, J., Seamone, C., Baines, M. "The Ocular Manifestations of Sexually Transmitted Diseases." *Canadian Journal of Ophthalmology* 1990; 25(4): 179.

Gill, J., Arlette, J., Buchan, K. "Herpes Simplex Virus Infection of the Hand." *American Journal of Medicine* 1988; 84: 89-91.

Klotz, R. "Herpetic Whitlow: An Occupational Hazard." *Journal of the American Association of Nurse Anesthetists* 1990; 58(1): 8-13.

Shaw, G., Langston, A. "Herpes Simplex Virus Encephalitis: The Need for Early Diagnosis." *North Carolina Medical Journal* 1986; 47(1): 17-18.

Taylor, P., Nozik, R. "The Patient with Conjunctivitis." *Hospital Medicine* 1992; 28(8): 24-46.

Whitley, R. "Herpes Simplex Virus Infections of the Central Nervous System: Encephalitis and Neonatal Herpes." *Drugs* 1991; 42(3): 409.

Whitley, R. "Herpes Simplex Viruses." *Virology.* Second Edition. Ed. B. Fields, D. Knipe, et al. New York: Raven Press, 1990: 1867-86.

DIAGNOSIS

Ashley, R. "Laboratory Techniques in the Diagnosis of Herpes Simplex Infection." *Genitourinary Medicine* 1993; 69: 174-83.

Ashley, R. "Inability of Enzyme Immunoassay to Discriminate between Infections with Herpes Simplex Virus Types 1 and 2." *Annals of Internal Medicine* 1991; 115: 520.

Ashley, R.L., Wald, A., "Genital herpes: review of the epidemic and potential use of type-specific serology." *Clin Microbiol Rev* 1999; 12(1): 1-8.

Fairley, I., Monteiro, E. F., "Patient attitudes to type specific serologic tests in the diagnosis of genital herpes." *Genitourin Medicine* 1997; 73: 259-262.

Koutsky, L., Stevens, C., Holmes, K., Ashley, R., Kiviat, N., Critchlow, C., Corey, L. "Underdiagnosis of Genital Herpes by Current Clinical and Viral-Isolation Procedures." *New England Journal of Medicine* 1992; 326(23): 1533-9.

Verano, L., Michalski, F. "Comparison of a Direct Antigen Enzyme Immunoassay, Herpchek, with Cell Culture for Detection of Herpes Simplex Virus from Clinical Specimens," *Journal of Clinical Microbiology* 1995; 33(5): 1378-9.

OTHER STDS

Centers for Disease Control and Prevention. "An Evaluation of Surveillance for Chlamydia Trachomatis Infections in the United States, 1987-1991." *MMWR* 1993; 42(SS3): 21-27.

Donovan, P. "Testing Positive: Sexually Transmitted Disease and the Public Health Response." New York: Alan Guttmacher Institute, 1993.

Institute of Medicine, Division of Health Promotion and Disease Prevention. *The Hidden Epidemic: Confronting Sexual Transmitted Diseases.* Eds. T. Eng and W. Butler. Washington DC: National Academy Press, 1996.

INDEX

NOTES

MANAGING HERPES

NOTES

MANAGING HERPES